The *birth* of Magdalena

A Personal Journey Towards Healing in Three Trimesters

MB ANTEVASIN

Cover Design: Michelle Fairbanks, Fresh Design
Interior Design: Alexa Bigwarfe of Write.Publish.Sell
www.writepublishsell.co

Published by Kat Biggie Press
ISBN: 978-0-9994377-5-9
2nd Edition Copyright © 2017 Mb Antevasin

Library of Congress Control Number: 2017
First Edition: June 2011

10 9 8 7 6 5 4 3 2 1

PRAISE FOR
THE BIRTH OF MAGDALENA

"This book contributes to the discourse on women's birth experiences and how powerful they can be, both negatively and positively powerful. "

~*Tisha Graham CPM, CCE, CD, CLC*

"A brilliant voice in the darkness, Antevasin brings extraordinary insights that provide a healing path for mothers everywhere who find themselves in unhealed trauma, yet having to hold tight while they parent their own children. Relatable, raw, and full of wisdom, we find ourselves uplifted with hope and a new, powerful way to gracefully hold both the beauty of motherhood and the unexpected gifts that it can bring."

~*Oceana LeBlanc*

This book is a shining example of the power of women to transform themselves with their ability to walk through the flames toward healing from within. The author's willingness to open completely to the vulnerable place necessary to share her own raw process is such a unique gift. She offers her own experience as an inspiration for others to follow their own path to a more authentic and whole self. There is nothing I love more in my midwifery practice than to see exactly this sort of transformation. Michelle has truly taken her own inner work to a new level in order to offer it up to the world.

~*Heidi Ricks, CM, LM*

Dedication

This book is dedicated to the women in my family,

the women who have become my family,

and the women that find inspiration in this book

while they are on their own journey.

Blessings on your journey!

♡MB

Contents

Acknowledgements

This book would not have been possible without the circle of *seven* extraordinary people surrounding me with their love and support and the baby who took this journey with me.

I would like to thank my husband with whom I have found unity, identity and purpose,
my sister who will always be my best friend,
my bold, beautiful daughter,
my two gentle and amazing sons,
my inspirational midwife, and
my doula who came into my life
right when I needed her, and who continues to give me guidance and nurturing.

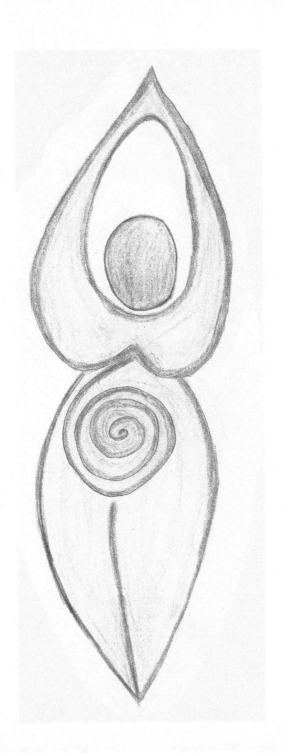

Preface: The Conception

Here I am, sitting at the kitchen table talking with my grandmother with the sun shining through the big picture window, and all of the beautiful birds flocking to the birdfeeders out back. Grandma is angry. I have heard this birth story countless times, and despite being over six decades later, the disappointment and hurt is still palpable. We have all these sayings about how the birth of a baby is the happiest moment in your life, but that is reserved for small talk. In reality, birth is powerful and scary and hard. Overcoming our fears and finding our strength helps us to become mothers, and birth can be beautiful, inspiring, empowering, and joyful. But all too often it is stripped of that, and we are left with something much less. Our power is taken from us. Like my grandmother's birth story, the violations and the traumas go unacknowledged and thus are carried with us because we are not given the opportunity to heal.

My grandmother was the youngest of a large family, with the babies all born at home. Her mother (my great-grandmother) would labor at home with her mother-in-law who was a nurse, and when it was time, the doctor would be called to the house. He didn't use any drugs or instruments, and only needed to use stitches once after a breech birth. Just over twenty years later, my grandparents were building their own house in the woods when her first labor started. She was taken to the hospital where her doctor attended births and she was given a nice private room. When her water broke, she tried to get out of the bed and go to the bathroom to clean herself up, but the nurse wanted her to stay in the bed. The injection is the last thing that she remembers from her first birth. That is all she ever says about my mother's birth.

It is her second birth that comes to mind more often. She tells me about how much pain she was in when she woke up screaming and strapped to the bed. She was glad that she could only get a shared room that time, so that she had a roommate to hear her cries and come save her. When the nurses came in, they could not even tell her if she had given birth to a boy or a girl, since the babies were on a different floor. When they finally brought her son to her, she said he looked like he had been in a fight. She had gone to a larger hospital that time because she had placenta previa and had been bleeding towards the end of the pregnancy. The baby had the umbilical cord wrapped so tightly around him that he couldn't descend, so they must have used forceps, but she does not know the details, because she was not conscious for the birth, and they did not tell her much afterwards. But she was cut wide open, and even 60 years later, still complains of trouble using the bathroom. It hurts me to sit with her and know that she has not yet healed from these births, physically or emotionally.

Three decades later, my mother was part of the social movement for natural birth and breastfeeding. At her first birth she had been given Demerol and Scopolamine which they call "twilight sleep." She doesn't even like to get Novocain at the dentist because of how it makes her feel. She won't drink more than one beer or glass of wine because she doesn't like to feel like she is losing control. She says that she was drugged at her first birth because the nurses were uncomfortable with the noises that she was making. She says they didn't take the pain away, she still had plenty of that afterwards, but what they had taken from her was her memory of the birth, which she can never get back. At her next 3 births, my father was charged with protecting her from the nurses so that she could labor how she needed to, and "moan like a cow" if she wanted, but most importantly, she wanted to remember.

By her fifth birth, she chose to labor in the pool.

This was long before they started offering water birth in the hospital; she just stayed home in the backyard pool and floated. My father sent us each out in turn to try and convince her to get out of the pool and go to the hospital. She happily floated there all day, squeezed into an inner tube and gently floating in circles around the pool. When she finally got out and called the doctor, he asked her to meet him at the office where he took one look at her, and then they all drove quickly down the highway and into the parking garage of the hospital. Eleven minutes later my youngest brother was born. My father tells a funny story about how as they were running down the hallway, the nurses just thought that he was a hysterical new father and they tried to get him to stop and fill out the paperwork.

I knew that when it was my turn to become a mother, that I would have a natural birth, even if I had to be on guard against the system. I knew from all the media reports that many women were now choosing epidurals or elective cesareans, but I chose natural birth. I read a lot of books, I chose a midwifery practice and I signed up for Lamaze classes. I took my prenatal vitamins and I never missed a prenatal appointment. I practiced breathing and made a CD of music for labor. I went to La Leche League meetings and was excited to become a mom but I was a little nervous about breastfeeding.

I didn't know of any professional birth doulas in my area, but my friend and I had read about them in magazines. I was the doula for my friend's first birth, and she would come to help me at mine. I had my mother there to protect me and my loving husband for support. When labor roared the loudest, I just held on to my husband and sang, and sang, and sang. It was the hardest thing that I have ever done, but I was doing it. So, as I lay on the operating table desperately trying to see my birth reflected in the stainless steel above me, I couldn't help but wonder how this had gone so wrong?

I too, had become a mother in America. Who could conceive of such a thing? But I didn't want to be sitting with *my* granddaughter someday, still broken and still in pain. I wanted to heal. I wanted to bring birth in our family back to where it was a century ago. When/if my daughter gives birth, I want it to be one of the happiest moments of her life. This is what motivates me to keep trying. This is what keeps me going when it is hard. This is why I take another step, even though sometimes I can't see the path. And this is why I share with you this story about my journey towards healing.

This is a birth story, but even if you haven't given birth and maybe never plan to, birth is such a beautiful image for the process that we go through when we need to create something new. And when we undertake something huge like saying that we are going to heal the intergenerational trauma for our family; it helps to be able to see the milestones as you progress through the phases. Sometimes we begin a journey before we can even fully conceive of what we are getting ourselves into this time. We move through the trimesters as an idea first takes shape, then changes and grows and as we transition it gets ready to be birthed into a new life. For me, the births of my babies were what woke me up, pushed me way outside of my comfort zone, made me find the courage that I never knew I had and shook me out of my delusions and into a new reality. Each of my births changed me physically, emotionally, mentally, and spiritually.

When I started this healing journey, I had no idea how much of ourselves we bring to our births. I thought that we could separate out the stories of what has happened to us, and who we truly are. I did not know how much we carry those stories within us and they craft our lives and weave their way into every thread of our families. Becoming a mother makes us look back at what brought us here, and makes us think about what we can do differently for our children. We want what is best for them. We look through our past with a fine toothed comb trying to find where we went wrong so we can save our children from the same kinds of suffering, but at the same time we need to forgive ourselves and others for what we didn't know then.

I also wanted to save other mothers from having to learn the hard way like I did. I started writing after attempting to have conversations with other moms. If you've ever tried this then you know that once you become a mom you may never again manage to finish an entire sentence, never mind a complete thought. I would have a mom ask me a question and then run off to save her kid from falling off the playground or take her kid to the potty and then I wouldn't ever get to answer it, and all those unanswered questions would keep me up at night. Or someone would make a comment that just didn't make sense to me, and before I could ask them what they meant by that, they'd be gone, leaving me to figure it out on my own. So I started to write (late at night or in the minivan during preschool if the baby slept) so that I could finish a whole paragraph or at least know where to pick up and finish my thought later. And maybe you can find some moments of quiet to sit and read this book and use a pretty bookmark to save your place if you need to put it down and come back to it later.

Another thing that kept me up at night (as if nighttime feedings weren't enough) was trying to resolve all of the discrepancies between how I felt inside and how I seemed to be perceived by others. One time another mother said that I was just "that kind of mom" who has a natural birth, and she just wasn't that kind of woman. But she didn't know that I had to go through a traumatic surgical birth, and then a really painful VBAC to finally get to my peaceful homebirth. One mom said that I had so much courage, but she didn't know that I was terrified the entire time and never really felt like I was doing anything right. Sometimes, someone would say that they were surprised about something that I always thought was really obvious, like when I told a woman at the office that she didn't have to apologize for talking about prayer and she explained that she never thought that I was spiritual. Another time, a woman in my doula group said that "the energy that you use to birth a baby is the same energy that you use to make love." The way that she said it you just knew that she was picturing a candlelit room with gentle music and roses and someone looking at you with love in their eyes. She had no idea that sometimes both sex and birth can be an entirely different kind of experience, and I didn't know how to make her understand without shattering her beautiful image. But then I also looked into the eyes of a woman who had only ever had abusive relationships and traumatic births and I told her about how she could have an empowering transformation and then I held her in my arms while she labored under soft lights and danced to gentle music and birthed her own baby into the world with love and power and joy.

I feel like sometimes we put other women up on a pedestal and think that we can never be like them, and never have what they have, and never do what they have done. We say that they are just lucky, because we can't see all of the steps that it took them to get to where they are now. We see something that in our hearts we know we really want, but then we put the idea of it out of reach because we don't think that it is attainable, so we don't even dare to want it. We believe that we can't have it, so it is better to not even try than to feel rejected. If we tell ourselves that we don't deserve to be happy or healthy or loved, then we don't feel as disappointed when we don't have that in our life. We rationalize to save time. I would just say "my body hates me" to sum up why I had so many symptoms that nobody could explain and was in pain everyday. I just knew that something was wrong with me and that I was un-loveable and so it made sense that people would hurt me or reject me. But when I held my baby in my arms and felt true love and true joy and true power, I knew that I needed to tell a new story.

I started to gather my notes and I reflected back on how I had gotten to this point. I thought of how many years it took before I was able to hold my baby in my arms. I thought of how amazing it was that I was even here to write. And I thought about how complicated and messy it all is. I find that I don't do a good job of fitting neatly into just one box. I want to pick multiple choices on the quiz because there is something of value in each one and they are all right in different ways.

I wonder how you are supposed to choose just one dessert off the menu when they all sound so good. So I realized that there is no way to come up with a magic formula for birth or for motherhood that would work for everyone. There is no equation. You can't calculate it. There is no right answer. I had gotten caught in the trap of perfectionism where you hide everything that is not perfect and you are so ashamed that you can't ever forgive yourself. So even though I love school and the dream of finding the right answer and I had set out to write a how-to book with all of my notes, I found that I was being called to share my own story.

And then after my last birth, as my doula and I sat drinking tea and talking about how much I had learned on my mothering journey, she said that I had to write a book (and I take homework assignments very seriously) so I called her nine months later and told her that I was ready to birth my book.

I share my story with you on these pages so that you will know that you are not alone. This is the story of my healing journey. I know that word is used a lot nowadays, but I don't use it lightly. I say "journey" because it was no walk in the park. At times, I didn't know how I would find the courage to keep going, but in the end, it was all worth it. It took me three tries to have my empowering and healing birth. It took me many years to understand what I needed to do to start healing. I know that I can't take the steps for you, but I will leave some breadcrumbs on the path for you to follow as you take steps on your own journey. I will share with you some things that helped me to make connections and see the patterns so that I could start to heal my family stories and so that I could avoid passing on my wounds to be healed by another generation. Sometimes it's frustrating when I finally find something huge that was hiding in plain sight the whole time, and maybe this will help you to find something in your own story that was there all along but you never understood the significance.

So even though I have always felt that it was safest to hide, I will let you see how this strong, courageous woman carries a hurt little girl inside and is just pretending to be the perfect mom who has it all figured out. When we break the silence, the secrets no longer make us sick. When we speak our truth, it helps us all to heal. I will walk ahead and shed some light on the path for you. So, if you will journey with me, I will take you through the three trimesters of growth and change that it took for me to finally transition into healing and birth a new story.

Chapter 1: A Good Girl

Be a good girl. How many times have I heard that phrase in my lifetime? It seems that I have always strived to live up to that expectation. I am always trying to make everyone happy, and I am scared of disappointing anyone, especially my parents. They never really needed to discipline me, if they so much as looked the least bit disappointed I would fall apart. But after all of this molding into everyone else's image of who I should be and what I'm supposed to do, it makes it even more difficult to discover who I truly am, or what I want for my life. I feel like I am always trying to make sense of how the world sees me and why it doesn't seem to match who I am inside. They say that to heal you are supposed to speak your truth, but I feel like sometimes we carry so many stories inside of us that it can be hard to know how all the pieces go together.

In school, I always tried my best and did what I was told. I was terrified of my teacher and even more worried that I would make a mistake. I vividly remember one day in First Grade when I knew the answer was correct, but the teacher had marked it wrong. We had to write the first letter of the word for the object shown in the picture. I had written a T for "taxi", but apparently in the part of the country where the worksheets were made they are called "cabs." When I stood up for myself and dared to question the teacher and her answer key, I was called "fresh" in front of the whole class. I was so ashamed at having been labeled despite all my attempts to be a good girl. It was my most important job in life, and I had failed at it already.

That was to be only the first of many such stories throughout my childhood. I wanted to please everyone, but since that was impossible, it didn't make for such smooth sailing. Looking back, it seems silly to think of the little things that mattered so much to me in my childhood. In the grand scheme of things, and in light of all the suffering in the world, I know that I had a privileged childhood. I grew up in a safe neighborhood where the kids played outside and rode their bikes after school. I had two parents who loved me and read me bedtime stories. We always had dinner on the table and Santa Claus remembered to come to my house every year, and we always hung our stockings in the same place, and baked the same cookies from our family recipes. I had a new doll for every birthday and my mother showed me how to sew clothes for them. My Dad built me a special shelf that was big enough to hold all of my porcelain dolls and took me to the store to pick out the perfect shade of green (Lime Fizz) to paint the walls of my new bedroom. We hung the shelf over my beautiful new bed where I could sit, wrapped in my grandmother's quilt, and say my prayers and count all of my blessings.

So now you know why it seems so ridiculous to talk about how life isn't perfect, when I was given so many opportunities that I know others never had. But even when your life is full of so much goodness, one dark secret can be like letting a single drop of ink fall into your glass of sparkling water, and soon your whole world turns black. It can become hard to remember your blessings when it seems like there is a darkness staining your whole story. Even my happy memories seem to have this undercurrent of shame. If only I had known then that my soul could be washed clean, that the dark sediment would settle to the bottom where the sludge could be removed and I could pour off the clean water and start again. I wish someone had told me sooner that it was possible to heal. And I'm sure that so many people tried along the way, but I just couldn't hear them at the time. I wish that I had realized that I was never meant to carry it alone. But those were all lessons that would come with time. And in the meantime, I was just a little girl, trying to find my way in the world.

I desperately wanted to make friends with the girls at school, but I always felt like I couldn't do that without hurting my mother. My mother didn't approve of the latest fashions or wearing make-up. She was from the generation that had fought hard to rebel against those shackles, but I just wanted to fit in. I went to the Catholic School, so we all wore the same plaid uniforms, but everyone would find little ways to look "cool." The other girls had the fancy binders with pictures of kittens and unicorns, and they would carry them through the halls with pride, but I had to make do with my plain, old folder. Mom finally let me get a jean jacket, but it was dark blue denim when all the other girls were wearing stone-washed. The popular girls wore nail polish and eye shadow and had designer purses. I put on nail polish at a slumber party once, but I couldn't relax and enjoy myself because I was so afraid that my mother would find out. But in the world that was my suburban American elementary school, my worst crime was that I couldn't even do a cartwheel. So I wasn't allowed into the Unicorn Club and I had to play football with the boys at recess. But apparently, I threw like a girl.

I did have a "best friend" growing up, which means that there was a girl my age that lived in our neighborhood. She went to the public school, but we'd play in the afternoons and have sleepovers on the weekends. Unlike me though, she had lots of outfits in the latest fashions, and even got her hair cut and permed at a salon. So, obviously, since she was more sophisticated, she would always get to choose what and how we played. If it was dress-up or dolls, she would get the prettiest outfit and then I would choose next, since I didn't care anyway, or so it would appear. Even worse, I usually had to play the boy.

One day my mother went to a craft fair at the church and came home with something pretty for me. She had bought me a pair of barrettes that had green and gold ribbons braided through the metal and then the ribbons hung down long and flowing with my hair. I was so proud and I went to show them to my friend. She ripped them out of my hair and took them and buried them in the dirt. It still hurts when I think about it. And that is probably why I decided that I didn't need anything pretty. When I was older someone said that it was cool that I didn't care about being pretty. Ouch. Of course I cared, but I didn't dare show it.

It amazes me to look back and realize that despite all the ways in which she made me miserable, I would have done anything to be her friend. Her rejection was worse than anything she did when she played with me. Every day after school and all weekend I would do what I was told. But regardless of how hard I tried to please her, if she had anyone else to play with, I would be discarded. If one of her friends from school came over, she would pretend that she hated me and deny that we were friends. But I knew that I was really her "best friend" because I was the one who kept all her secrets.

Worse than the days when I had to play the boy were the days when I actually got to choose the pretty dress-up clothes, or the beautiful doll. On those days my doll would have her clothes torn off and would be raped by the boy doll. Or I would have to undress in front of her and she would make fun of me and make me do things I didn't want to do. Looking back, it seems wrong that a girl that young knew about such things, but I think that even then I understood that no matter how badly she was hurting me, someone had hurt her much more. Her other friends never knew the real girl. She seemed so strong and confident and dominant, but she was the one who was really vulnerable. And though I was probably her one true friend, it was dangerous for her to have someone who knew her secrets. And because I kept those secrets, I knew that I would never really be able to be a good girl, and no one could ever really love me.

When I went to the public high school, the school was so much bigger and there were so many new people. I wanted to be friends with some of the new girls that I was meeting, but I couldn't really, because all the nice, smart girls that I enjoyed being with couldn't possibly really like me. I couldn't ever be myself with them, because they would stop liking me. But who was I really? Who was the real girl? Was it the girl who was always trying to be a good student and the Girl Scout who liked to help people or the girl who was secretly broken? So I never could really fit in anywhere, because I never knew who I was.

Growing up, there were so many mixed signals. I wanted to be beautiful, and I wanted to fall in love and live happily ever after. But I was taught at home that beauty and fashion are not important. My mom wouldn't even shave her legs or wear a bra like all the other moms. But she taught me to be modest and cover my body, especially my private areas. I felt so dirty and ashamed of my body, but then I was just supposed to change my clothes in front of everyone in the locker room for gym class or right out in the open at the town pool while my mom just held up a towel. I felt like all of my bodily functions were dirty. I would die of embarrassment if I thought someone could smell me. I remember the shame I felt in 4th grade when I farted in class and everyone knew it was me. I was so mortified at the pep rally in 9th grade because I had my period and

I could smell it, so everyone must know. I never went to another pep rally. I would rather skip school and risk being caught.

And what was I supposed to make of all those mixed-messages about sex? The beautiful, popular girls were sexy and everyone knew it. They got all the attention from the boys, and all the girls wanted to be friends with them. But good girls don't have sex. Good girls save it for marriage. Sex is for making babies. Sex is something that men want, and women are supposed to play hard to get. But I wanted a boyfriend. I wanted someone to pay attention to me, to ask me to dance. It was exhilarating the first time a boy touched me at the back of the school bus where nobody could see. I would let the boys touch me, hoping that they would want to be my boyfriend. But it was always the same; they would do what they wanted, so long as no one could see. I was not the type of girl that they would date, or kiss in public. And I was a good girl, I was saving "it" for marriage, so what would be the point of dating me?

And then I met a boy who really understood me. He was so smart and we were lab partners in biology class. I felt like I could be myself with him. I liked myself when I was with him. But we also had a friendly competition that pushed us both to work harder and get better grades. He was my first *real* friend, and since he was a boy I had fantasies of marrying him when we were older. He was the first person that I kissed because I really wanted to, and it was magical. I was happy for the first time in my whole life. It was a great feeling, if unfamiliar. But he was not the same race or religion as we were, and my mother said that he was nice but we shouldn't date. His parents didn't approve either and he said we should just stay friends. I was devastated when he broke up with me.

But the good news was that it was a new year and I had a new friend to turn to during this crisis. There was a girl I knew from church, and we had chemistry class together. We wrote notes to each other all day at school and folded them into little triangles and passed them in the hall between classes and then talked on the phone every day after school. She took my side against the world. She asked me to hang out with her outside of school, and to go out with her for her 16th birthday. All the popular teenagers would spend Friday nights just walking around the center of town in groups, and I was finally going to be included. It felt so good to finally be one of the cool kids. As we walked, a group of older guys started to follow us and flirt with us. We flirted back and started walking together. My friends latched onto the good looking guys and I hung back, but their friend paid attention to me, and that felt good. When we ended up at their apartment, we sat and talked on the couch while some of my friends went into the bedrooms. He asked my name, but I wouldn't tell him my last name. It was fun to flirt, but I never planned to see him again. After I left, he got my friend to tell him my name, and he looked me up in the phone book and showed up at my house the next day.

I tried to avoid his calls and his visits, but he was persistent. I had wanted a boyfriend for so long, but now I was nervous. I was still in love with my biology lab partner, but it was kind of flattering that someone really liked me like that. He told me what I wanted to hear. He said that I was beautiful and sexy (which seems kind of funny now when I look back at pictures of a skinny kid with freckles and knobby knees), and my friends all said that he treated me like a princess. The girls were all jealous that I was only a sophomore but had an older boyfriend who was already out of high school. I talked about him at school and I thought that it would make my lab partner jealous, and make him realize that he really wanted to be more than friends.

So, the white, Christian man came to my house to ask my parents for permission to take their 15-year-old daughter out on a date. He didn't own a car, so my father would drive me to the school for the basketball game, and I would meet him there. I was glad to be at a chaperoned event at the High School where the teachers would make sure that nothing happened. But after my father drove away, my date told me that we were going to leave the game and walk to his apartment downtown. I tried to tell him that the teachers wouldn't let me leave the school, but then they just told him that we couldn't get back in to watch the game if we chose to leave. I had been playing the roles that I had been given for so long, and was used to always doing what I was told, that I didn't know how to say no to him. I wanted him to be happy and to be my boyfriend. When we were alone in his room I told him that we could kiss, but that I was saving "it" for marriage. He told me that he understood. He said he respected that. He said he loved me. But he was pulling my clothes off. He said he just wanted to look at me because I was so beautiful. But then he was on top of me and he weighed more than me, and I couldn't make him stop. It was like the nightmare that I'd had since childhood where there is something heavy pressing on my chest and I can't get up and I can't scream.

And then it was over. It was all over. I couldn't pretend to be a good girl anymore. I couldn't save "it" for marriage and no one would ever love me. I would never live happily ever after. I was ruined. So what could I do? In that moment, everything just stopped. I stopped eating. I stopped sleeping. I stopped going to school. I stopped trying my best. I was gone.

After that night, I told him I didn't want to see him, but he would come to my house and knock on my window after my parents were asleep. He refused to leave, and I was afraid he'd wake my parents, so I let him in. What did it matter anyway? I was already ruined. He used my body so many more times after that night, but the damage had already been done. I tried to pretend that it was romantic, but it didn't feel like love. I kept hoping he'd stop. I couldn't sleep because I was so afraid of that knock on the window. But I was scared to make him angry, because then he would just hurt me more. He would make me do things that were so disgusting and degrading, but then he'd be so nice. I lost track of what was real. I lost track of myself. I tried to tell my parents so many times, but I didn't know how. Their disappointment in me would hurt even more than anything that he could do to me.

Anyway, once the baby came everything would be better. I had always wanted a baby. And besides, he'd said that he would marry me. And even though I had planned to go to college and I couldn't imagine marrying him, I figured that was my only option now. He'd shown me the ring at the mall, and he was saving up to buy it for my birthday. My birthday was spent in tears, because a single red rose is not a diamond ring. My godparents had sent me a "Sweet 16" necklace, but it just made me cry because I knew that I wasn't really sweet, and it broke my heart to think of them finding out the truth. And then my girlfriends called to say that they were not coming to my birthday party and to tell me about how much fun they were having somewhere else. They were upset and they took it personally that I had become so distant. He had been keeping me all to himself, and there was no "me" anymore. There was nothing that could have prepared me for a relationship with someone so manipulative and controlling. But I was only dating him because my girlfriends had told me to, and I had just wanted them to accept me.

And then he went missing too. He had moved out of his apartment and I had no way to reach him. His roommate said that he was living in another town with a woman who had her own apartment. I rode my bike to his work to tell him that I was pregnant. I knew that would bring him back to me and fix everything. I practiced how I would tell him as I pedaled my bike up the hill. I practiced exactly how I would say it, and how he would react with surprise and then joy. I never imagined that he'd be mad. He was so angry that I had shown up there. And then when I told him, all he said was, "So." I rode back down the hill in tears. My whole body shook, and that night, the baby flowed out of me with the tears. When I flushed the toilet, I knew that I was truly alone.

Even after we broke up, I couldn't sleep. I was terrified that he would show up and hurt me again. I tried to talk to my mother, but she said that he broke up with me because men only want one thing, and he left because I wouldn't give it to him. So, that conversation left me even more confused. My mother used to tell me about how she always checked in on me at night, and how she loved to watch me sleep. I knew that she was lying because that would have saved me so much pain. Each night, I kept hoping that she would catch him there and then my father would be so mad that he'd do something terrible to this man that had hurt his little girl. I kept waiting for my father to be the hero and save me.

One night a few months later, the police came to ask my parents about him. The neighbors had called the police because they had seen him outside our house at night and they were worried. I thought that finally my parents would wake up and realize what had been going on, but they told the police that he was a good guy and that we'd been dating. But the fact that the neighbors had seen him outside my house recently only terrified me more. I kept thinking of him outside my window, watching me sleep, and I would panic.

I'd walk around in my house all night, double checking the locks and looking outside, and listening for a knock on the glass. I'd call the only person I could really talk to about this. My lab partner was my only real friend, my first real boyfriend, and the only person who really saw me and heard me. He was the only person who had ever loved me for who I was. And although we weren't ever going to be a couple, it gave me strength to know that he understood. And it was good to have a friend to talk to while I shivered, alone in the darkness. He lived far away now, so it helped that he was still awake at that hour, but it only made him feel helpless that he couldn't hold me and make me feel safe.

After a long summer of crying and walking alone and making mixed-tapes of sad songs, I started to hang out with my girlfriends at school again. They set me up with a boy from our school bus who said he liked me. After dating a man who couldn't afford a car and was working manual labor instead of going to college, it seemed like a step-up to be asked out by someone who lived in a big mansion and drove a fancy car. We had been dating a couple of weeks when he asked me to go to the Junior ROTC military formal dance with him, and I wore a beautiful long pink gown and I felt like a princess. But after he picked me up, he didn't drive me to the dance. He said he was too embarrassed to be seen with me in front of his friends. He took me to his house, and he took my dress off and he did what he wanted with me. That night I had my first "episode." I collapsed in a heap of pain with a terrifying combination of severe abdominal pain, a splitting headache, and an asthma attack all at once.

My mother took me to all of the doctors. I had a colonoscopy and a laparoscopy, but there was nothing visibly wrong. I woke up from surgery hoping for an answer, but they said that it was nothing. I was fine. But I did not think it was fine to feel debilitating pain like that. They couldn't diagnose anything, but I got put on birth control pills, painkillers, migraine pills, and a bland diet. Nothing worked. When I collapsed in the hall at school, they called an ambulance. The doctors at the Emergency Room couldn't find anything either, and when they pulled my pants down in front of my friend to give me a shot of pain medication it accomplished nothing.

I was already trying to handle all of these things that were way beyond my years. But then a series of events really put me over the edge. It seemed like everything happened at once. My friend who always drove me to folk group practice at church died suddenly from a stroke and it was shocking because she was only in her 40s. Then in the same month we had to go visit my great-grandmother because she was dying, but she didn't remember me anyway. I had been visiting her regularly for my entire life and I was always trying to please her, but she was never impressed by my efforts. While I played the piano for her, she would tell the other nursing home residents about someone else who came to visit who could play beautifully. But I kept trying. They say that things come in threes, and after her funeral we got the news that a school friend that I'd known since First Grade had killed himself. Much like me, he had found some solace by escaping into heavy metal music, so it was a final insult that he had to wear a preppy turtleneck to his funeral to cover the bruising. I still remember how my feet were frozen to the ground when I tried to turn and walk away from his grave, and I don't think it was just from the freezing temperatures. This was just about the time that my baby should have been born. Everything seemed so surreal.

After that I was trying to figure out what life is all about and why we are even here. Then my little sister went into the hospital for emergency brain surgery. They had found the brain tumor just in time, but if they didn't operate that day it may kill her. She had only thrown up at school and failed her eye exam in the same week, so it was good that my mom knew that it was unlike her and followed her mother's intuition and brought her in right away. I took my little brothers to the neighbors' house and tried to keep them happy playing with other kids while I was freaking out inside. The next day I couldn't go to school. I couldn't sit there as if nothing was happening, so I skipped school and played pool with my friends all day. The guy with the pool table hadn't gone to school much anyway after his older brother hung himself. I went to visit my sister when she woke up, and seeing her so tiny and hurt in the Intensive Care Unit was the scariest thing I had ever seen. But I put on my brave face for her and I tried to brush what was left of her hair as I choked back my tears. Once she was put in her own room, I tried to go and play games with her to keep her busy. But she was too angry to play and threw the board at me. She blamed my mother for making her have the surgery. She was too young to understand the alternative. She hadn't felt that sick, and then the doctors had hurt her with invasive surgery and excruciating spinal taps. She stayed mad at my mom for years.

I had been so scared, and I was so grateful and so relieved that she had lived. So how could I say what I was really feeling? I missed my sister. The little girl that used to laugh and sing and brighten all our lives was gone. She had changed and was like a totally different person. I still loved her and I always will, but there will always be an ache in my heart for my little sister who waved goodbye that day and then never came back.

Then, one day that summer, the phone rang. I knew something was wrong before I even walked in the room and saw my mother's face. It was like when there is a storm coming and you can sense it before it hits. It was my aunt on the phone, and they were talking about my cousin, the one older girl in my family that I looked up to more than anyone else. It wasn't just that growing up with all those boys, she was my only female cousin. She was my role model. She was such an amazing person and I always tried to do everything just like her. I kept waiting to be older so that we could be best friends. Now she was dead. She had taken a break from her graduate research and gone on a trip and died of a virus that nobody had even heard of before. I tried to brush what was left of my sister's hair to cover her scar, and even though it was now summer, I put on the black velvet hat that my cousin had bought for my birthday, and we went to another funeral.

It seemed like all of my hopes and dreams for my future had died. I started wearing all black and smoking cigarettes and I drank whatever liquor we could find in our parents' cabinets. I escaped into my music and I wrote poetry. I finally became more popular though. No one wanted to be my friend when I was an A-student and a Girl Scout who dreamed of becoming a saint. I was much more fun to hang out with when I didn't care about the consequences.

Since I was getting invited to all the good parties now, I met a guy who was a bass-player in one of the local heavy metal bands. We had a mutual crush that grew into something more over a semester of gym class together. He was a great guy and he loved me even when I told him the truth about my other relationships. He didn't think that I was ruined. He thought that I was smart and beautiful. He took care of me and he was the one person who would never hurt me.

But when I finally went off to college, I really wanted to start over. I wanted to be able to find my true self again and break away from all that had happened. Relationships are hard enough, but living in a different state made it harder. My boyfriend was so afraid to lose me and he kept pulling me closer. He was a mess without me, and he loved me too much. I was trying to move forward and he kept pulling me back. He loved a "me" that I didn't want to be anymore. Breaking up with him took more strength than I knew I had. I shook and I sobbed and I begged God to fix it. But God told me to let him go. I had been praying my whole life, but in this moment of surrender when my heart was aching and I was grieving so deeply, I heard the voice of God speak to me so clearly that it shook me to my core. God said that everything would be okay. God said that he would send someone even better. And then I went off of the pain meds, I went off the bland diet, and I started to sing again.

I spent a summer away from my parents' home, and away from my college. I took a job up north at my favorite place where we had vacationed every summer in my childhood, and when I wasn't working I would sit by the lake and think or I would swim alone all the way across the bay. I biked all over the island, and I became physically strong. I began to find myself again. But then after my new boyfriend from college came up to the lake to visit and waited until after we made love to tell me that he had been cheating on me, my coworkers picked me up from the middle of the road where I had collapsed, and drove me to the hospital. It was actually in that small, country emergency room that a doctor first called them "episodes." Pathetic as it may be, that was the best description I'd gotten, even after seeing all the medical specialists for years. Anyway, it was obvious that I still had a ways to go towards healing my wounds. But if someone had given me the answers then, I don't know if I would have learned as much, or healed as completely as I have in the long-run because I was able to do the deep work and discover the answers myself.

When I returned to college for the fall semester I found a flyer taped to the back of a door in the bathroom stall in the Student Union. I started talking to a woman at the rape crisis hotline on the phone every few nights. She helped me to find the courage to speak out. Deep down I was still a good girl, and I couldn't live with myself knowing that the man who had raped me when I was in high school may now be hurting someone else because I never spoke up. I know that other people had hurt me as well, but since this man was older, it meant that it was clearly wrong without me having to go into too much detail and without feeling like I had to prove anything. I drove back to my hometown and I filed a police report about the statutory-rapes that had occurred when I was 15-years-old. Once I was back at college and had some distance between us, and with the support and encouragement of my sorority sisters, I somehow found the strength to call my mother and tell her the whole story.

I had started the teacher-training program that semester and there was a cute boy in the program with me, and from the first day I knew that he was the *one*. He walked me home the first day and talked about how he believed in helping people and how teaching would work so well with raising a family. He could see the real me, and he liked me as I was. I liked who I was when I was with him. I could see a future with him. I told him the whole story about why I had to travel to my hometown in the middle of the semester, and he actually went with me to the court for the hearing. I had written a letter to submit to the judge. I only wanted to know that this man wouldn't be able to hurt anyone else, and I felt that jail time would only make him more violent. He got a suspended sentence which meant that he had to go to therapy each week and talk about what he had done, and if he missed a session then he'd go to jail for ten years. He also wasn't allowed to leave his state, which meant that I could finally sleep at night without worrying about him stalking me again, looking in my windows as I slept. I was shaking with fear and was sick from having seen him again, but I walked past him and out of that courtroom, and into my future. I tried to leave that hurt girl behind me and move on.

This cute boy was like the best mix of my biology lab partner and my bass-playing high school sweetheart, but he was so much more. He could see the real me that I had kept hidden from the world, and he still loved me. This time I got a real diamond ring and a church wedding with a silk gown that my mom and her friend helped me to sew, and a honeymoon that was actually enjoyable despite my fears. In this relationship that was equal and reciprocal, making love could be something that was pleasant and made me feel good. After all that I had been through, it felt like I finally had made it through to the other side. We talked about everything and we were truly best-friends. We started teaching science at a local school and we earned our Master's degrees and we bought an old farmhouse with a swing and a tree house in the backyard. We had big plans and bigger dreams and most importantly, we had each other. We were living happily ever after.

Chapter 2: The Illusion of Care

As I lay in my hammock looking at the sky between the leaves of the two maple trees, I prayed a rosary and asked Mary if it was finally my time to become a mother. I knew it hadn't been the right time when I was in high school, but I had still wanted that baby, and loved it so much. Every February I thought of the birthday that I should be celebrating. I counted the years and looked at other babies and then kids that would be the same age. And I waited. I had gotten married in the church and we had bought the house with the big back yard, complete with a tree house and a swing. We had finished graduate school and were settled into our teaching careers. I was finally ready to have a baby on my own terms, with the right man. I tried to be patient and wait the 6 months that they say it will take after going off the pill, but I was having erratic periods. The doctor said that I wasn't ovulating and tried using progesterone to bring on a period and get me to ovulate. My body had betrayed me again.

After waiting so long to become a mother, I was

having trouble being patient. But I wanted to do the right thing. The doctor suggested a pill called Clomid that would basically have my brain tell my ovaries that it was time to release an egg. I had been trying to have faith that I would become pregnant when the time was right, and I didn't know if this was considered cheating. I spoke to the priest about my concerns, and he thought maybe God was putting this doctor and this opportunity in my path, and that maybe I just needed to trust in God's plan. He said that there are no pills stronger than God. So, I took the pill and I bought an ovulation predictor kit and a home pregnancy kit, and I started charting my temperature every morning.

Any amount of charting and "trying" is hard on any relationship. It kind of takes the fun out of it. So we were glad to have something to increase our chances of getting towards our goal of becoming parents. I was started on one pill, and if that didn't work after 3 months, they'd increase the dose. I was so relieved when I first got that positive test while I was still on the first dose. I had read about so many couples who struggle for years and try so many things. I had had so many negative home tests that when I went for another check up and the doctor came in and said, "it's positive", I had said "for what?". I had started to think it would never happen, and the fact that I was pregnant took a while to sink in. But by the time I got to the car, I was already ecstatic. Just knowing that I could get pregnant was such a relief.

The fact that I was going to have a baby was still months away, but I was so happy and glowing in that moment. My mother was in town and had gone with me to the appointment, and on the drive home my mom told me not to get excited; but it was already too late. She talked about miscarriage rates when I just wanted to stick my head out the window and scream my triumph to the world. When we got back, I ran into my husband's arms and shared the news. I wanted to just stay in that embrace, in our own little universe, our family. At our wedding they had said that the two of us had become one, and in that moment it felt so real.

I had been preparing. I had read all of the pregnancy and birth books and had chosen to use midwifery care for the pregnancy and the birth after the medical doctor had helped me to conceive using the pharmaceuticals. Now that I was pregnant, I figured that my body would know what to do, and I was going to have a natural and beautiful pregnancy.

But when I started losing a lot of weight and feeling really sick, they wanted to check if I was having an ectopic pregnancy. I had an early ultrasound and they found that I had conceived twins, and I was losing weight because my metabolism just couldn't keep up with two growing babies. Either the Clomid or my letting go of the idea that there was a "right way" worked so well that I had released an egg from both ovaries. The doctor had briefly mentioned the possibility of having twins, but I think she said there was maybe a 6% chance. We like twins, they are so cute, and we just wanted to start a family. It wasn't until after we saw those two gestational sacs on the ultrasound that they started using the term "high risk".

After that, they began to feed me more and more fear at every appointment. They told me not to get excited, because chances were that both babies would not grow. I went to all my appointments and I met all the midwives in the practice, but I couldn't find support for the things that really concerned me. Like the fact that I was starving and couldn't seem to eat enough. I had a long commute and a lot of responsibilities at work because I was running a science education program at the University now, but I tried to find ways to take care of myself as I grew even hungrier and more exhausted by the day. I went to the nutritionist for help, and she told me to make stews and eat tahini. I was too tired and wasn't ever home long enough to make stews. And I had never even heard of tahini and didn't know where to buy it or what I would do with it if I found it. But I tried my best to be healthy for my babies.

I loved getting to know my babies over the months of the pregnancy. On one car trip, every time we hit a bump, Baby A would kick. Not long after that I could feel Baby B too. It seemed to make sense because at that very early ultrasound when they could see the follicle scars on both ovaries, and could measure the gestational sacs by the number of days, they had said that Baby A was conceived first, and then Baby B about a day later. When they started to be able to see the babies, they would measure them and make sure they were both growing, and after the first trimester, they were both about the same size. Now that I could feel them, I could really start to learn about their two very different personalities. I could tell when one was awake and one was asleep. It was usually that "Baby B" was trying to sleep and was woken up to play by "Baby A". "Baby A" was the dominant one, the boss. "Baby A" had gotten there first and set up shop, and told "Baby B" how things would be done.

I had a baby shower at our home, one at my school and one at my husband's school and then we traveled to another one that my mother-in-law hosted for us. We had everything ready because we knew that twins had more of a risk of coming early. I stopped commuting to work and I had hired a replacement to cover my maternity leave at work. I guess it was a good thing, because at 30 weeks, I started having contractions.

The contractions were regular, coming every 4 minutes. My husband was on the phone with his mother just making regular small-talk, and as I waited to use the phone, I charted the contractions. Over an hour later, I finally called the midwives and was told to come to the hospital in my town. I drove myself over and the midwives met me there and I was helped into a hospital gown and put into a bed and put on the baby monitor. My husband finally caught on that we were doing this and met me there explaining that he couldn't leave the lasagna in the oven. They tried giving me Terbutaline and Magnesium Sulfate to stop the contractions. I was on the monitor for over an hour and I was scared. It was too early and the babies were too small. I talked to the babies and told them to stay in longer and grow bigger, but the contractions wouldn't stop. They wheeled me to the ambulance with just thin sheets and the gown between me and the winter air, and aside from freezing, I was embarrassed to be escorted by two male EMT's without wearing any clothes.

As soon as I was wheeled into the larger regional hospital that had a NICU, the contractions stopped. I was kept for a few days to be watched, but since I was no longer considered to be an emergency, the nurses would forget about me and I'd have to call on the buzzer and ask them to bring me food. I was so hungry that I couldn't wait for the scheduled meals and the nurses had to scrounge up extra food to keep me from starving. You'd have thought that there would be a nutritionist at the hospital who would know how many calories it takes to satisfy a twin pregnancy. At least the babies still had good appetites. And I still talk about how I even ate a sandwich with rye bread and Swiss cheese, which I hate, but it was all that they had. It was just another sacrifice that I made for my babies, and an acknowledgment of who was really in control here.

The hospital stay was also the beginning of a period of quiet loneliness. I wasn't used to sitting and doing nothing. I was used to having my students and other professionals to talk to every day. I was used to having goals and projects and deadlines. After a few days in the hospital bed, the doctors sent me home and put me on bed rest. I would get up from my bed in the morning, go to the kitchen, make a blender full of smoothies and pack a basket full of food, and then move into my recliner for the morning. The smoothies were my best idea, because I needed the calories, but I would get tired from having to chew so much. I had always loved to eat and I never thought that I would grow to hate it so much.

I was excited to be on bed rest, at first. I thought it would be nice to be able to catch up on my reading and get some projects done. I had a cross-stitch to finish for the nursery and blankets to crochet for the babies and it was nice to have someone substituting for me at my program so that I could focus on the pregnancy and think about being a mom. But then when the swelling began, I developed pregnancy-induced Carpal Tunnel Syndrome and the pain in my wrists made it so that I could barely hold a magazine, never mind a book. I certainly couldn't hold a needle, and I couldn't play any musical instruments because I could hardly feel my fingertips, or they would go all pins and needles. So much free-time, and it was all going to waste. I tried to finish the baby blankets, but crocheting one line at a time it was a slow go. I laid in my recliner, and ate and slept, and watched every movie that they had at the public library. I rubbed my enormous belly and I asked the babies to stay in there until at least 35 weeks.

After losing so much weight in the beginning of the pregnancy, I was making up for it now. I was now 50 pounds over my starting weight and my skin had stretched so far that it was now actually ripping open and bleeding if I reached for something. I was so swollen and sore and I had to be checked at the midwives' office twice a week since my blood pressure was so high. I had what they call Pre-eclampsia and I was ready to be done with this pregnancy and I wanted to see my babies. At 37 weeks I started contracting and my mother took time off from work to come be with me. She's a nurse, so this wasn't really time off for her because I needed so much care at this point. She would massage the fluid up my legs from my aching feet, and put my pants and shoes on for me so that I could go to the midwives' office for my appointments. I was 2cm dilated and 90% effaced. The babies were big enough and could come anytime, but they needed to come soon. My blood pressure was going up and my swelling had gone from extreme to ridiculous.

My uterus kept contracting all day, and I gained about two pounds a day of water weight. My skin was now so tight that it was shiny like a mirror, and it hurt so much. Even experienced Labor and Delivery nurses would come to stare at the freak. I wasn't having a very beautiful pregnancy, but I was still holding on to the idea of a natural birth. After two weeks of suffering, I finally started to let them talk about induction. They gave me one more weekend to try to go into active labor, and we scheduled the induction for first thing Monday morning. Now I wanted the babies to come out, so I went off bed rest and I walked and walked. I was so out of shape by this point from being in bed for so long that it was hard to walk. That, and I was humongous and in so much pain. But I kept going. I bounced up and down and told the babies that now it was time to come out. I had read that sex could bring on labor, and after having been banned for the last 5 months (to avoid having labor start too early), we tried it. My husband was a pretty good sport given the technical difficulties. I wish it had worked.

On Monday morning they started the Pitocin drip. Instead of a contraction every few minutes, they came right on top of each other with no breaks in between, and they were really strong. They gave me Magnesium Sulfate to protect my brain in case I had a seizure from my blood pressure being so high. That drug makes you feel like you are going to burn up from the inside and I was hallucinating. They broke my water and hooked me up to a contraction monitor and a heartbeat monitor for each baby. I had one on my belly for Baby B, but they inserted an electrode into Baby A's scalp to get a more accurate measure since that baby was coming first. The IV dripped, the machines beeped, and we all waited.

I was still trying to "go natural" even though that seems like a ridiculous notion at this point with all the wires and the beeping machines and the drugs. I didn't want any more drugs than they were already using, and I didn't want to numb the experience. My husband held me and my friend came and put cool cloths on my head and I sang along with my birth CD. I felt strong because I was doing it, and it was hard. I dilated quickly and was 6cm dilated by lunchtime. My husband put on his scrubs because twin moms need to deliver in the Operating Room. I was excited to see my babies soon, and even more so at this point, I was ready to be done.

No one went to get lunch because my labor was moving along so quickly. They checked me again and I was 8cm dilated. There was this one song that worked really well with my labor, and it was a perfect lullaby for my babies. My husband kept repeating that track on the CD because it seemed to be the only thing that helped. I sang my song, again and again and then it was dinnertime. I was starving but no one fed me. I kept enduring one contraction after another, but I was still 8, and 8, and 8. I knew I was going to die. My little brother came to stand at the foot of my bed to encourage me, but nobody else could see him there. The doctor told me that I could keep doing this for another two hours if I wanted, but she was going to do a cesarean after that anyway. Then Baby A's heart rate dropped suddenly, everyone jumped into action, and the doctor said, "no more discussion", she was doing it now. I was wheeled down the hall and the babies were cut out of me. I felt them being tugged out of me and I started to shake and cry and vomit.

When I woke up, I was back in a room. My mother stood on one side of me and my husband stood on the other side. They were each holding a baby to one of my breasts and I was nursing. I figured I could stop being nervous about nursing for the first time, and I went back to sleep. So, here I was, a mother. Finally.

So why is it that despite all the logic and the evidence before us, we continue to believe things that just aren't true? The images that we hold in our minds can be so ingrained that we cannot see what is right in front of us. We bring a lifetime of belief systems and values to every decision that we make, and pregnancy and birth is no different. When I had trouble getting pregnant, the doctor could fix it. As soon as she told me I was pregnant, then I could allow myself to feel the changes in my body. And as soon as I started going to my prenatal appointments, I believed that I was receiving prenatal care.

I had such a clear image of a midwife in my mind from the books that I'd read and the movies that I'd seen. I thought it was great that the obstetricians at my hospital had midwives in their medical practice. I went to see the midwives so that I could treat pregnancy as something normal and natural. But apparently that wasn't going to be possible as soon as they saw those two gestational sacs. I became a special case, high risk, anything but normal. They paid such close attention to me that I assumed I was receiving the best possible care.

I did receive the best medical care that they could offer. But what I really needed was what is called primary care or prevention. I needed proactive, not reactive care. In fact, I kept asking for it. I asked for advice on nutrition, since I ate constantly but still did not feel good. I ate three complete meals in between dinner and breakfast. I kept candy bars in my desk and in my pockets just in case the hunger came on suddenly. Even after seeing three midwives, two doctors and the nutritionist, I still had not found any advice that was specifically geared towards a twin pregnancy.

Despite the fact that every time I asked for help I was ignored, I still could not believe that they weren't taking care of me. They were doing what they are trained to do, which is to monitor and wait and see if I would need a medical intervention. The medical model is trained to step in when things go wrong, and then fix them. So at each prenatal I was weighed and measured and they checked my urine and took my blood pressure. And then when I could officially be labeled with pre-eclampsia they watched me even more. I still assumed that they would tell me what to do to be healthy, but they just waited until it got worse and worse and then when I was near death they put in an IV with pharmaceuticals to protect my brain, but they still did not cure anything.

When I started having contractions and my cervix

started to efface and dilate, I knew that I would start to see the midwifery care that I had read about. I knew that she had a few tricks up her sleeve and she would pull them out anytime now. I started to see one of the midwives almost every day, practically begging them to *do* something, anything. Nothing was progressing. Basically, they were waiting for me to say yes to an induction or to surgery. I didn't realize at the time how little control they had in that practice, with every step being watched and supervised by the obstetricians. And for the OB/Gyn's, surgery was their idea of doing something. I knew that midwives could help with positioning and I'd read about them even reaching in and turning the baby if they needed to do that. I had had an ultrasound to check the babies' positions and sizes, but no one gave me any information that would help my labor to progress.

After two weeks of trying to push that early labor and unproductive contractions into active labor that actually opened my cervix, I was admitted to the hospital and put on pitocin. I felt like such a failure. They even broke my water for me. I had been walking in public places thinking of how funny it would be when my water broke all over the place and how everyone would freak out like in the movies and TV shows. But that never happened. They hooked me up to all of their machines so they could watch the strip of paper instead of asking me how I was doing. They made me stay in the bed so that they could get good data for my chart. The only problem was that I hadn't even been able to lie down in my own bed for months. I'd been living in the recliner 24-hours a day since my ligaments couldn't stretch enough for me to actually lay down. They couldn't move the hospital bed into any position that was comfortable, so I ended up leaning over the tray table with a pillow on top. I was catheterized because I couldn't pee when I was in so much pain. They did countless internal vaginal exams throughout the day.

I worked with a very painful labor in that really uncomfortable position for over 10-hours. For all those hours the midwife sat at the foot of the bed. She never touched me to comfort me. The doctor was there because I was high risk, and the midwife had no power when the doctor was there. A week before, in the same practice, a twin had died at birth and the fear of the staff was palpable. I made it to transition and was hallucinating and thought I was going to die, but still the baby did not move. I begged the midwife to reach up in there and do something, but she did nothing.

Everyone watched the monitors. But it was better than when they looked at me. They had taken my clothes and I was mostly naked, except for that little tube top over my abdomen that held the monitors, and two gowns (one in the back, and one in the front) that barely covered my body that was like a beached whale, just trying to survive. They kept making negative comments. As soon I had walked in, a nurse had called out "Whoa, what a uterus!" But I'd have thought she'd seen plenty of those. I realized I must look really bad. Then there was a lot of discussion about how huge my bladder looked since I could neither get into a position to use a bedpan, or pee in front of an audience. They all marveled at how shiny my skin was since it was pulled so taut, but no one could make it hurt any less. One nurse even mentioned that I had a lot of pubic hair, and I wondered what that had to do with anything. Pardon me for not worrying about grooming parts of my body that I couldn't even see anymore.

If I mentioned that I was in pain, or that the Mag Sulfate or Pitocin made me feel horrible, they would ask me if I wanted to die. Worse was when they asked me if I wanted the babies to die. I assumed that my entire purpose in going to the hospital was so that they would prevent both of those occurrences, so aside from coercion and torture, I couldn't see any reason to keep asking me. I assumed that as medical staff they would want to hear information about how I was feeling, but I was quickly shut up any time I said anything. I didn't feel as if I was welcome there, they were solely interested in my uterus and my cervix, and my being there was just a nuisance and a distraction.

After six hours with my cervix dilated 8cm, the doctor told me that she was going to perform surgery, basically whether I liked it or not. I didn't want to consent, but it wasn't really a question anyway. And then conveniently, the machine beeped and the doctor was saved from trying to be polite to me or having enough of a conversation for me to give informed consent and she could just go into emergency mode and be the big hero. I looked over to my mother, desperately trying to get her to save me. I had brought her with me because she had given birth five times, and she was the one who had told me the stories and given me the books about natural birth, so she would understand. She was a nurse, but she was also my mother and it was her job to protect me. I needed her to do something, *now*. She was still angry about how they had treated her at her births, and she had talked about having to advocate for yourself against the system, but now after working as a nurse she had been trained for too many years to follow the doctor's orders. I think she was one of the half-a-dozen people that it took to get my body flipped over and into position leaning over the back of the bed. It was actually kind of comfortable once I was there, and the baby's heart rate returned to normal, but the anesthesiologist was already getting ready to insert the needle for the spinal anesthesia and the doctor and nurses were already prepping for surgery.

After they pushed me quickly down the hall like a big float in a parade, they left my family outside the door. Then the nurse held me in her arms so that the anesthesiologist could work on my back. She had one of those big, comfortable bosoms like those ancient statues of the Great Earth Mother, and it felt so good to be held by her. And the anesthesiologist was so gentle with me and he talked to me like I was a person. I think it was the first time someone said something nice to me all day. I was craving a little loving touch and human kindness, and it made the horrible situation almost bearable.

Then they laid me down and tied my arms off to my sides, like I was being tied to a cross, and my husband and mother joined me in the operating room. They had already started, and I tried so hard to watch what was being done to me on the other side of the screen. I could see them make the incision in the image reflected in the stainless steel light fixtures above me. I was amazed at how much I could feel. I couldn't feel the cut of the knife, but I felt them pulling and tugging on my insides. I felt them pull the baby out, and they held her up to the side quickly, but someone stood between us and I missed my chance to see her. Then they said that I had a son. I knew the babies were off to my left somewhere, but then I started to feel sick as they pulled on my innards. And I think my body was in shock at having been separated from the babies so abruptly. I remember puking before I blacked out.

I woke up back in the room and I was nursing. I had planned to have my mother there to help, and she made sure that the nurses brought the babies to me right away. We had talked about it before, and I was glad that the babies were able to get what they needed, but I was a little sad that I couldn't even hold them. And I was horrified to wake up topless with strangers in the room and the door wide open. Waking up and finding my body being used was difficult for me, even if it was my own babies, and I had asked them to do it.

Over the next few days I was kept in the hospital for more medical care. I was medicated for the pain and they changed the dressings and checked my incision. When they took my catheter out, I had to get up and walk all the way across the room to use the toilet. That was the longest, hardest walk of my entire life, but they practically yelled at me for complaining about the pain. There was not enough strength in my arms to hold that pillow to my stomach hard enough to avoid feeling like everything was going to fall out. I just wanted to lie back down, but they said that I had to walk to heal properly. I tried to take a shower because I felt so gross. I woke up to the smelling salts and a nurse I'd never met standing over my naked body, with the door to the hallway wide open.

I had waited so long for them to get here, and I just wanted to take care of my babies. I wanted to help change their diapers, but I couldn't stand up long enough. I sat in the chair for a little while in the new bathrobe that my Mother-In-Law had given me at my baby shower and I felt almost human for a moment. My husband would change a baby, and then bring them to me to nurse. I had friends and family come to visit. They wanted to see the babies, but it was hard to play hostess when I felt so horrible. I didn't like having to breastfeed in front of an audience when I was just learning how. There was important news on the TV and everyone assumed that I would be interested, but I was in some other world. And mostly, it was hard to be with people that were happy and excited when I just wanted to curl around my empty, wounded belly and cry.

Chapter 3: Welcome to Parenthood

"Y ou'll never sleep again," they'd say. How many times had I heard that during the pregnancy? Everyone tries to warn you, but how do you prepare for that? In college after you pull an all-nighter to study, you get to sleep after the test is over. If you party too much or stay up too late, you can make up for it the next day. Until you become a mother, it is hard to envision taking on a job that is 24 hours a day, 7 days a week, for basically the rest of your life. You think that someone can take the babies and let you sleep, not realizing that the ache of their absence will be so physically strong that you still can't rest. And even if you manage to drift off sometime in the next few decades, it will never be anything that resembles the sleep that you had before you became a mother.

Right from the start we were exhausted. The labor was so long and intense; I had used up all of my energy. My husband hadn't wanted to leave my side, and he hadn't slept or eaten in days. He didn't eat breakfast before we went to the hospital because he was too anxious, then I was so close at lunchtime, then they were born at dinnertime, then we were parents. By the next day he was ready to collapse. Everyone else had gone, but he wouldn't leave me to go home and sleep, especially because I could not get up out of bed to get the babies, and I couldn't hold them by myself. The nurses offered to take the babies to the nursery so that we could sleep. He finally fell asleep on the chair and I wanted to let him rest. I couldn't sleep because I could hear my babies crying down the hall. I was panicking. I was shaking and nauseous. The nurse gave me a pill but it didn't help. Finally, they brought the babies back to be fed, and when I held them in my arms, the sick feeling went away. It happened again the next time. Every time that they took them away I would get physically sick. The medical staff treated the symptoms, but they did not seem to understand what I really needed.

The babies were both born at over six pounds each, with perfect Apgar scores and no evidence of distress after all. They were perfect except for the little scar on the side of my daughter's head by her ear where they had screwed the electrode into her scalp. They had Band-Aids from where they'd taken blood for their newborn screening tests. They had identification anklets so that no one would confuse them with someone else's baby. I was the only one who could tell them apart. All the visitors said they could only tell them apart during the diaper change, it was the favorite joke. But, they were two totally unique babies. One was pink and one was yellow. One had a square face and the other heart shaped. And they had totally different voices and personalities. But, everyone was in awe of how big and healthy they were. I had the perfect little family. They say that's all that matters. They say I should be grateful.

I went home before I was ready. After four days at the hospital, my husband wanted to be home in our own house and to sleep in our own bed. My mother had already been visiting for three weeks and she had used all of her vacation days, and she had to go back to work the next day. She wanted to help us get settled at home before she left. I would probably never feel ready anyway, so I agreed to go home, even though my insurance would have covered one more night. After all that, I couldn't go upstairs to our bed anyway since I was recovering from surgery, so they set everything up downstairs. I sat in my recliner and my husband lay down next to me on the couch and we each held a baby. We were exhausted, and we were alone, and when we both collapsed there was no one else there to take care of the babies. We had fallen through the cracks.

Family and friends came to visit. We took pictures of each person holding the babies, since we knew it was all a blur. If it wasn't for those pictures, I wouldn't even remember who had visited. I hate the pictures of me though, I was so gross since I couldn't step into the tub, or stand long enough to shower even if I got in there. I was exhausted and in pain and still huge. They told me to put towels under me when I went home, since the water from the extreme swelling and the IV fluids would all start to leak out. It was pretty disgusting to just sit there and have so much sweat pour out of me. But I was happy when the swelling went down and my feet and my hands and my face went back to something that resembled my former self. I also had to wear pads for the bleeding and a bandage for the incision. It was an awkward time to entertain guests.

Newborns nurse about twelve times a day. So, I had about 24 feedings a day. They were just learning how to breastfeed, and they'd been through a lot and they just wanted to snuggle, so they would nurse for about 30-45 minutes. Then I could go pee or grab a snack while my husband changed the diaper. Then I'd do the same with the other baby. We had charts for feedings and diapers since it was all a blur. I had a chart for my pain medication and set an alarm since the 4-hours would pass without us even noticing. While I cuddled and nursed I could take a little nap in my chair for a few minutes at a time.

After "giving us a few days to rest" (ha!), more family came. It was right in time for my milk to come in, and now on top of everything else, I was hugely engorged. My little 34B push-up bra had already been replaced with an industrial 40D sports bra, but now that didn't fit because I had more than enough milk in my breasts for twins. Before my body had time to adjust and regulate the supply to something realistic, the skin on my breasts tore and bled because it couldn't stretch anymore. While the babies were being entertained by their grandparents and aunts and uncles, I snuck into the other room to use a breast pump just to soften the breast enough so that the babies could latch on. Otherwise, they'd just beat their angry little faces against this huge rock, unable to get the areola into their eager mouth. But the pumping just encouraged the breast to make more milk, and it was a vicious cycle. At least I now had a freezer full of milk just in case. When I finally found a moment to cry to my mother on the phone, she convinced me to give up the pump and she explained how to push inwards with your fingertips to soften the areola so that they can latch on, and then after a few more days of that my milk supply finally regulated and the engorgement wasn't as extreme.

The problem with help is that plenty of people offer, but they don't necessarily understand what is really needed. My family tried to give me a break by taking the babies in the other room. I could hear them all talking in the kitchen and having fun without me. They didn't know that I felt left out and lonely. And they didn't know that I couldn't sleep anyway since I was getting physically sick again, the same as when they took the babies in the hospital. I wished they would just sit and talk with me in the living room, but when I called to them no one could hear me. I was in too much pain to get up and go to them, so I just sat alone in my chair and cried.

My husband was allowed two weeks of paternity leave from work. By the time we got settled at home there was already one week gone, and then the second week was a blur. My aunt offered to come and help for a week when he went back to work. I was getting used to nursing and the engorgement had settled down. I had finally showered and I slept in my own bed for the first time in months. I could finally enjoy having company, and she sat and talked with me and I loved hearing all the family stories. I was beginning to enjoy being a mom and felt like I was joining all of the other women in my family.

And then my third week at home, after my aunt

left, I started to feel worse. It happened gradually at first. I had been trying to wean myself off of the pain medications, because I didn't want to become dependent on the narcotics. So I had taken a little less each day. Then I noticed that I had been gradually increasing the frequency, and then the dose. I was back on the full dose again, and then they weren't even working. I was in too much pain to lie down, and I started sleeping in the chair again. I couldn't stand up long enough to change a diaper at the changing table. That's how my mom found me when she came to drop off my grandmother who was planning to stay with me for the week.

We left the babies with my 80-year-old grandmother and my mom drove me to the midwife's office. I sat in the rocking chair, freezing and sweating and shaking. There were happy pregnant women and new moms with their babies. I remember sitting in that same waiting room before I got pregnant, thinking how wonderful it would be when I was one of them. But here I was, miserable from the pain and the fear. I thought I was going to die because it just kept getting worse and even with the drugs I had severe abdominal pain and a really scary fever over 105°F. After waiting over an hour like that, my mom finally went to the desk and explained a little more forcefully this time that the babies were home with my grandmother and I had to get home to feed them.

My grandmother could give them some the expressed breastmilk with a dropper, but my breasts were filling up and I needed to get home.

I finally saw the midwife, and she called it a uterine infection. It was so bad that they wanted to put me on IV antibiotics, but I could not be readmitted to the maternity ward. I could check in to the sick floor, but I could not bring my newborns with me. How was I supposed to heal if I was engorged and separated from my babies? I knew that I would feel worse being separated from them and hooked up to a breast pump instead. At almost two hours away, my breasts were rocks, I was miserable and I just wanted to go home, so they gave me more pills and sent me home. For the next few days as my fever stayed over 105°F, my grandmother took care of the three of us. I was barely conscious, but she would burp and change the babies and bring them to me to nurse. I was so disappointed because for years I'd been trying to get Grandma to visit so that I could show her my yard and my town, and she was finally here and we couldn't even leave the house.

Eventually the fever broke and I gradually got better. When spring came I took the babies outside and put them in the double stroller and we went for walks, first around the yard, then down the street. I would bring them out on a picnic blanket and we'd watch the clouds go by. I sang and they cooed and kicked their feet, and the two of them would roll to be closer to each other, and when they held hands my heart would melt. After five months in the big blue chair it felt so good to be outside again. We even started to go out to town, and I'd put them both in the ring-sling and carry them from the car to the library or the park, and then put them down on a blanket to play. My chubby little bundles were already getting heavy.

After all that my body had been through, it was an accomplishment just to feel "okay," but I was hardly back to normal. My ribs were still spread about six inches further than usual and my hips were wider. I had a herniated diastasis so large that I could put five fingers across the hole in between my abdominal muscles. When the babies crawled on my lap their knees would go right into my stomach and intestines because there was no abdominal wall there to protect them anymore. My feet had actually shrunk two sizes after the swelling went down, and I still can't get any explanation for how they lost length like that. I had numb areas all around my scar and itches that I couldn't scratch from the nerves all reconnecting. I had incontinence and bladder pain and hemorrhoids, and sex was excruciating. My whole body had been affected by the pregnancy, and it would take a long time before I even somewhat resembled myself.

I tried to discuss all of these complications with the midwife, but I was told that's just how it is, get used to it. I was told that the diastasis might get smaller with time, but the muscles would never knit back together. She ran a test for a urinary tract infection, even though I'd had numerous UTI's in the past and I told her that that *wasn't* what I was feeling. I explained that the pain that I was feeling was inside, in my bladder and that after I went pee it would hurt inside for about 20 minutes. I asked if there was some way to check if something was wrong from my surgery. I had had that infection, maybe something was left in there and was bothering my organs, maybe it was scarring, I didn't know. I asked about it on multiple visits, but no one would even discuss that there might be complications from the major abdominal surgery that they had performed.

When I read the statistics on the number of complications from cesarean sections, I wonder how many other women are not even being counted. I requested a copy of my medical records, and reading through the notes made me so angry. "Patient sys she's hungry." "Patient says she's having contractions." And my favorite: after two weeks of prodromal labor and swelling over two pounds a day, they wrote "Patient still uncomfortable." Can you say "understatement?" But the worst was that there was no mention at all of the severe infection that I'd survived after the surgery, and no mention of my other complications, it just said that they checked my urine. A few years later I wrote to the Medical Malpractice Board at the State Health Department, describing how they had lied on my medical records. They replied that what I received was considered the "standard of care" and that no further action would be taken.

So, where had I gone wrong? Was it my fault for assuming that the medical system was in place to take care of me? I thought that I had done my part in waiting until I was old enough, married and educated and financially prepared. Then I had done the right thing and gone for prenatal care, taken childbirth education classes and the tour of the hospital and read all the books. I had kept up my end of the bargain. My mistake was in having this image of a doctor who would "do no harm" and a midwife who would advocate for me and help me with nutrition and positioning and be there when things got complicated. I thought she'd be interested in my health history, and that she'd take care of me. I wanted her to hold me during labor, and help me when the baby had trouble. I thought I'd be able to go back and show her my big chubby growing babies and they'd have this bond because she was at their birth. I had wanted so badly to believe, that I had clung to this image and was blinded from the truth that the system had changed so drastically.

We now have a system where the "standard of care" has nothing to do with what is best for moms or babies or even midwives. The certified nurse midwives are not given the time, or the resources, or the autonomy that they need to actually practice midwifery. It was bad enough that I had this experience in which I was victimized and abused and ignored. The fact that it was done by people who were supposed to take care of me made it so much worse. The fact that they think it is okay to treat women like this and call it medical "care" is an outrage.

As if new motherhood isn't hard enough, you begin the hardest and most challenging weeks of your life physically and emotionally exhausted. Even if you manage to leave the hospital without physical scars or emotional wounds, you are probably exhausted and unsure of what to do. And then you are either thrown into a world where you need to get used to being out of work and home alone, or you need to figure out how to go back to work and be a mom at the same time. Or like many women, you find some new combination of the two that has no resemblance to your former life. Every decision you make impacts someone else, whose life is dependent on yours. Along with all the little joys comes an awesome responsibility. Nothing in your life is the same, and yet everyone wants you to just snap out of it and go back to normal as if nothing has changed.

So there I was, thrown into this new world of motherhood. I was sad to discover that the social mom scene is much like the cliques in high school. I could find different groups of women to hang out with, but I was often uncomfortable. It seems that there is so much competition to be the perfect mother. There is this iconic ideal portrayed in our media and ingrained in us so deeply that we can't fight the urge. I needed to make all these choices, all the time. I needed to be a "good mother". But then if you make what you think is a good, educated choice that will be best for your children, the other mothers think that you are judging them. Just because I made a choice that worked for me, that day, for my family and my situation, did not mean that I would make the same choice if I was in their shoes. I tried to assume that all the mothers were doing their best, whatever that may be. If they asked me for advice, or asked me what I did, I'd tell them, and I'd explain why I made that decision, and how it worked for me, for now. But I found that just like in school, no one wanted to be my friend if I was trying to be "a good girl," it was the same thing all over again now that I was trying to be "a good mother."

There are so many terms for everything now. One day my babies were playing on their quilt, and someone said, "Oh, that's great that you're doing tummy time." I didn't know that putting them down to play was so official. And the fact that I thought my sling was pretty, and it was so convenient that I could carry both babies and a diaper bag without dropping any of them, meant that I was joining the "attachment parenting" movement. I chose to hold my babies when they cried, and I did not make them "cry it out." I really did believe in a lot of the same principles that the mothers claiming to be practicing "attachment parenting" claimed were the best, but I had close friends who were doing the opposite, and they were just as convinced that they were right. I guess it all stems from your belief systems and family background. A lot of people who saw the way we parented were concerned about the babies ever becoming independent. They claimed that they would still be sleeping in my arms in high school, or still nursing when they went to college. There seems to be this rush to be all grown up before beginning school, which now starts at only three years old.

I did choose to breastfeed, and luckily it worked out really easily for me, for the most part. I had read too many things about formula and all of the possible problems, and I didn't want my babies to touch the stuff. I wanted to be very careful and give them to best start, the best way I knew how. So I was committed to exclusively breastfeed them for the first months. I knew women who pumped so they could work or go out for a while, but pumping was a pain. I'd just go out for a few hours and then nurse them when I got back. Once they were six months old and started solids, they would have a snack while I was away and I could stay away longer. I met mothers who had tried breastfeeding, and then used formula when breastfeeding didn't work. Some mothers only used formula and had no interest in breastfeeding. Lots of mothers did a combination of breastfeeding, supplementing with formula, and pumping and storing breastmilk. Every time I chose to nurse in public, or the babies insisted that they could not wait and gave me little choice, I was making a statement, whether I meant to or not. In this culture it is no longer a question of just feeding your baby.

I had taken environmental health courses in graduate school, and had learned about all the chemical hazards we are faced with from an early age. Going into parenthood with that knowledge made me very careful about what chemicals the babies were exposed to on a daily basis. In addition to breastfeeding, I chose cloth diapers because I'd read way too many things about the effects of the plastics and chemicals in disposables. But

I used some disposables sometimes for convenience. I'd read that even if you used plastic diapers for most of the day, it was good to let the babies air out for a while, or use cloth at least once a day. I paid close attention to their rashes and discomforts with different brands of disposables, and different detergents that I used to wash the cloth diapers and baby clothes. In our generation, we grew up with so many plastic products, that we are used to that new plastic smell, and don't realize how dangerous it can be. Part of our modern ritual of setting up the nursery includes a fresh coat of paint, new furniture, new carpet, new toys etc. that are all off-gassing in a small space. In addition to the plastics, there are also pesticides and fungicides and other chemicals that are used in these products, and the baby is breathing those as well. There are lots of Green or Organic products on the market now which are healthier choices, but they are really expensive. If I had a choice, I would buy older hard-plastic products and used furniture and rugs that had had a chance to off-gas before we bought them. My husband painted the nursery months before the birth, while I was out of town, and aired out the room thoroughly. I tried to think through every little decision, make the best choice I could at the time, and I had to assume it was better that not trying at all.

I didn't want to use cribs for many reasons, one

being the sheer square footage that a crib takes up, and especially the fact that most of the affordable cribs encased their mattresses in soft plastics that would off-gas into the nursery. We found baby hammocks online, and they were a good compromise. It provided someplace comfortable for them to sleep, and they were small and portable and made of cotton. They hung from a spring, so that when the babies stirred, the motion lulled them back to sleep. The babies slept great in those, but I never slept, I just nursed one baby and then the other in the rocking chair all night while my husband slept. I finally gave up on getting up and down all night, and decided that if they wanted to nurse at night they could come in my bed and nurse while I slept, laying down. Now I was in the "co-sleeping" movement. When had motherhood become so political?

Suddenly, I found myself in a world that was extremely complicated, and I was faced with countless numbers of choices each day. And, to make it worse, these are not choices about just my own life anymore. These are choices that will affect my children and their future. If I let them eat that food will it make them sick? If I let them play with that mean kid will it help them grow, or affect them emotionally? If I let them watch TV will they be at a disadvantage? And the media was always happy to present all sorts of horror stories and mother-guilt pieces for mothers to lose even more sleep over. As if I needed more reasons to stay up at night worrying. And when you finally leave the house to seek out some company and support, and then feel like the other mothers are watching you and judging each choice, that doesn't help either.

Entering motherhood for me was much like starting high school or college or a new job. I was leaving the familiar and heading into unknown territory, which was both exciting and terrifying at the same time. It can be a great opportunity to start over, to redefine myself. I figured that as long as people could see that I put my children first, that I loved and cared for them, that they would know the most important thing about me. I found some mothers that I had a lot in common with. We had children the same age and we were in some of the same attachment parenting and natural parenting and breastfeeding and co-sleeping groups. I thought that we could be great friends and maybe raise our kids together and grow closer over the years. Trying to make new friends is a little too much like dating. And like dating, comes with a lot of mistakes and heartbreak. In the long run, the real friends were the ones that stayed loyal and didn't judge me regardless of what I chose. The ones that I met because we had similar interests rejected me as soon as I made a choice that did not fit their model of a "good mother."

When I was at home with the babies, I had met some mothers that I thought could be good friends, but as soon as I talked about going back to work they protested. I had co-workers who had babies and went back to work at six weeks, and they were mad that I'd taken a year and a half off from work. Our other friends who didn't have kids stopped inviting us over, because their get-togethers were "no kids, of course." There is obviously no way to please everyone. Luckily once you have children your priorities change. Now, I mostly wanted to protect my children, and make sure that I was doing whatever was best for *them*. I put up with a lot less crap now. I have always put up with people being mean to me, but I don't want my kids around that, so I just get up and walk away. I tried to listen to my babies, and if something wasn't working they would let me know, and I'd try something else.

Right about when the babies had their first birthday, they started getting more mobile, and getting into everything. We moved everything to higher and higher shelves, then upstairs, then to the attic. We put up gates and plugged the outlets. But still, the two of them would have ideas about pushing the envelope, and they'd get into trouble. I found that I was yelling all day, and we were all miserable. So I took one room and made it totally childproof, and filled it with toys. Finally, I could sit and read a few pages while they played happily. It was worth stopping and thinking and making the changes so that we could find something that worked for all of us.

Once I felt like I had almost gotten good at mothering *babies*, now I had *toddlers*. Although it was challenging and exhausting to have newborns, it was easier in some ways. When they were babies, they cried when they needed something. If I met their needs, they were happy. Sometimes (okay, usually) I had to try numerous things before I got it right, and I was often frustrated. But then suddenly they had all these things they wanted to try, like running into traffic, climbing up high and then jumping off, chewing on random things like bugs and radiators, and other scary things. And now I found myself saying "no" all day long. They were exploring their world and testing their boundaries. Now it was my job to set limits and keep them safe, but still let them learn to be themselves and find their place in the world. I had to begin the process of letting go.

I had been putting so much pressure on myself to make the right choices, and keep them healthy and safe. Now I needed to do that, while letting them make some of their own choices as well. I'd let them play in a larger area, going in two different directions, choosing their own playground equipment, playing in their own way. I would hover somewhere in the middle and try to watch them both. For 99% of the time, things are fine. But then it seems like everything always happens at once. While you are running one way to catch one that is falling, you will lose sight of the other one and they will wander too close to the parking lot. If you stop to talk to another mother, you will turn to see what they are doing, and they will be gone from sight. They have a way of finding your blind spots, so that if you look quickly, they will both be hidden from sight, behind a slide or behind someone's legs. In that split second your heart sinks in your chest, you stop breathing and a million thoughts go through your mind. Then it is all fine, they reappear, and you go back to your day at the park. But I think that all of those stressful moments have a way of getting to you over time.

When I ran out of unpaid leave and it was time to return to work, it was so hard to think of leaving them for the whole day. Was I ready to let-go that much? Was I ready to trust someone else to make all those little decisions that add up to a whole day of mothering? But, ready or not, it was time and I had found someone that would be perfect. I had a long commute to work, and so I had a lot of options for daycares and babysitters. I wanted a home daycare or a smaller center, and I called every one between home and work, and there were none with two openings for children under two years old. I was talking over my frustrations at my attachment parenting group, and there was a mom who I had become good friends with, and she was looking for a way to stay home with her child, while still bringing in some income. She actually approached me with the idea of having my children stay with her during the day. We worked out all the details, and I was really excited to have found such a great solution. I felt like they would have the advantage of still being with a "mom" during the day, even if it wasn't me. She would play with them, and give them healthy snacks and lunches, and they would have another kid to play with. I felt like there were a lot of things that I didn't do as well as I would like, and she always seemed like such a perfect mother, so I thought this would be good for them.

When I first went back to work it was a huge transition. I figured we all needed time to adjust. I was so thankful that they were still nursing, so that we could reconnect as soon as I got back to her house. I also thought it was a good way for me to visit with my friend, and talk about how they had done during the day. That worked for a while, but then I started to feel like she was ready to be done for the day by the time I got back, so I started taking them home and then nursing. I was missing my committee meetings at work because she would call and have me come get them early. I started to leave work as early as possible, and usually picked them up at least a half an hour before the agreed upon time, because I felt like three children was wearing her out. I was now making decisions to try to please my friend, as well as my children, and my work was suffering.

At first it was just one thing here or there, but then all the little warning signs started to add up. I would have to take them home and sit them in a bath to soak the poop off their bottoms at the end of the day. She always said that they had just pooped, and she didn't have time to change them, but why were there so many unused diapers in the bag? By winter I had to soak their faces too because she couldn't wipe their noses for them. She seemed annoyed that they needed so much care, but they were the same age as her child, so what had she expected when she suggested this arrangement? She was being paid to play with them and wipe their noses and bottoms, and whatever else they got dirty. I started to notice behavioral changes in the babies as well. My daughter began to have worse and worse tantrums and my son was having nightmares. I read all the parenting books, and the consensus was that the "terrible twos" were coming early. Even though I felt like it should be her job, I tried to find solutions that would make it easier for her during the day, but she seemed mad that I didn't have any suggestions for ways to make them behave.

We finally had to call it quits when everything got to be too much. In hindsight, it is all so clear, but it was hard to see it while living in the moment. I had kept trying to find ways to make it work, and I really didn't have any other alternatives for childcare. The babies were miserable, my husband and I were miserable; the babysitter seemed miserable but wouldn't say anything. We should have taken the children out of there sooner, but we had no other daycare. I had called every place again, and there were no openings. If we could make it one more month they would be two years old and there would be alternatives. I am still blaming myself for not acting faster. But, until we made the changes, we didn't realize how much it was affecting them. When she finally lost it and quit, she literally threw my children out the front door, and our friendship went with it. I had a friend of the family who offered to watch them for a week or two while I sorted out daycare. After one week in her house the tantrums stopped, the nightmares stopped, and the rashes on their bottoms went away. The fact that I was trying to find a solution that would salvage our friendship, instead of just getting my babies out of there, still haunts me.

After that, it became clear that I couldn't ever let that

happen again. I couldn't put myself, or my friendships, or my family, or my career before my babies. They were totally depending on me, and I had let them down. I still had no daycare, but my husband and I took turns taking days off when my friend couldn't take them and we made it work for a little while. But it wasn't really working. I wasn't able to focus on my career. I wasn't able to get anything done at home. And, I felt like a horrible mother. I felt like I had waited and waited for so long to become a mother and now I was missing it. I had been trying to force myself to let go, and let them grow and become more independent. But things have a way of working out. The answers are there if we look for them. I should have learned by then that there is no one else that can give you advice or tell you what the right choice is, you need to trust your intuition, and know that when it doesn't feel right, you need to make a change. I still needed to remember to listen to my babies; especially now that there were three of them.

The Second Trimester

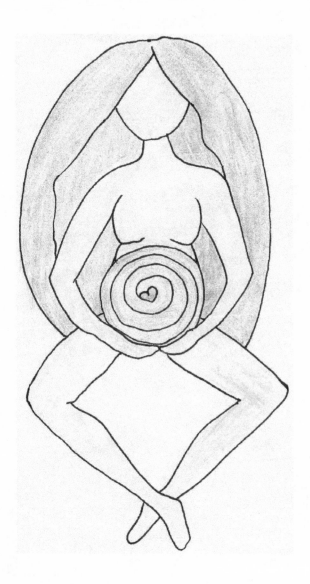

Chapter 4: Birth on My Own

With my next pregnancy, I tried to do things differently right from the start. We had wanted to just let things happen and we hoped that I would get pregnant without having to "try" so much this time. The wondering and waiting each month can wear you down quickly and can put a strain on any relationship and we didn't want to go through that again. When the twins were 18 months old I had gone back to work. They were still nursing all evening and at night, but as soon as I was away from them during the day my period returned. It was a pretty intense one, heavy and with severe cramps. When I bled again 28 days later I was so excited, because I thought that maybe I would be regular, finally. When I was 15-years-old and having trouble with irregular periods the doctor had said that I would probably be regular after my first pregnancy. Then he put me on "the pill" for ten years.

I thought that since I had a regular period, maybe

now I would be able to ovulate and conceive easily. But the next month, nothing happened. I was sure that I was just irregular again. I felt sick and started to worry that something was wrong. Maybe it was fibroids, or cancer. Then everyone got sick with the stomach flu. Everyone at work was sick and I had my hands full with two sick toddlers. I had been nauseous before everyone else got it, and I was still sick once everyone else got better. I had missed my period another month, and although I felt like I knew something, we didn't dare to even hope that it had been that easy.

I felt pregnant, but I couldn't trust my own feelings. We couldn't bear another negative pregnancy test, so we kept putting it off. Even when I was pregnant with twins, the home test had been negative. I started to notice more and more signs, but my husband didn't even want to get excited. As I changed one day I noticed that the saggy twin-skin on my belly had gotten taut again. Then I felt the baby moving. That Friday, after I had to pee for the 3rd time after getting home from work, I decided it was time to pee on the stick. For the first time ever, I had two lines! I put the cap back on the stick, put it in a pretty gift bag and hung it on the door handle for my husband to find when he got home from work.

On Monday morning I called for an appointment with a new midwifery practice. I had to go to a hospital

45 minutes away, since the one in our city didn't allow Vaginal Birth After a Cesarean (VBAC). It worked out anyway, since that hospital has a birth center with large rooms where you can labor and then stay in the same room for postpartum, and the midwives were much more independent. I only had to meet with the doctor once since I was a VBAC mom, and he would be on-call in the hospital during my birth, but would only be called if he were needed. I told the midwife about when I had missed a period, and when the conception must have happened. It wasn't hard to narrow it down, since I had two toddlers sleeping in my bed, and we didn't often have a babysitter. I had been too afraid to be disappointed, and too afraid that something would go wrong, but I had felt pregnant all along and I knew exactly how far a long I was. But when I told the midwife that I felt the baby move, she ordered an ultrasound, because I had felt the baby at 10 weeks, and the books say that you can't feel the baby until you are at least 18 weeks along. I went to the ultrasound to prove that I was right, but also to be reassured that everything was fine, somehow I didn't feel like I deserved to be so lucky.

I was right about the dates, and at that point, I had completed my first trimester and everything was perfectly alright. Even better, we didn't feel like we needed to wait to tell anybody since we had already put off that first trimester. And, the best part was that I was already feeling better, great actually. I looked great too. I had a cute little pregnant belly and my skin fit again. I had become super-thin because I was burning so many calories from nursing twins and trying to keep up with twins, and my twin-skin hung off of me. I was able to gain some weight despite the early nausea, so now I was just getting into normal sizes again. It kind of felt good to be able to sit on a chair without having to put a pillow under my bony-butt. And this time I was just gaining weight in my belly, hips and butt, not in my face and hands and feet! For the first time in my life, I really felt beautiful. I actually *was* glowing.

The hardest thing about the pregnancy was weaning the twins. I had a lot of friends who had tandem-nursed, so I just assumed that I could keep nursing toddlers sometimes, and nurse the baby too. In the fourth month though, I started to get sore. It happened gradually. At first I just started to notice that I didn't really enjoy nursing anymore. I would get irritated and hope that they would be done soon. Then my nipples got more obviously sore. Then my milk dried up and they would suck harder, trying to get something to come out, which became excruciating. I did my best to try not to cringe when they latched on, but I didn't succeed. They could tell that I was in pain, and we went from nursing eight times a day, to just bedtime in only two weeks. Then, two days before their second birthday, I lay down to sing them to sleep and neither one of them asked to nurse. I was relieved because I had been dreading it, but later that night I was so sad. They never asked to nurse again.

I couldn't believe how quickly it was over, and it was so hard to end that phase with the twins, but it did feel good to have a little time off before nursing the new baby. It felt a little like I had my body to myself again, which I know sounds crazy since I was pregnant. It also helped me to really start focusing a little more on the pregnancy. I started to get those pleasant second trimester hormones flowing and I got really horny. No one told us to abstain like they had with the twin pregnancy, so we had a lot of fun. It felt good to like my body. It was the first time in my life that I had a positive body image and really enjoyed being in my own body.

After not being able to find daycare for two, I gave up on the idea knowing that we'd never find or be able to afford care for three, so I quit my job. I knew it would be more than a maternity leave, so I took the time to interview for a really great replacement. My program at the University felt like one of my babies, and it was hard to watch it fall through the cracks when I was on maternity leave after the twins were born. I finally had gotten everything working properly again and it was hard to walk away, but finding someone to take over put my mind at ease. I left it in her capable hands and I turned my mind to preparing for the birth.

There's always this point in pregnancy where all of sudden you realize that there is this person inside of you, and somehow you are going to have to get them out. First you worry about getting pregnant, then staying pregnant, then dealing with the side effects of pregnancy, and then when you are feeling better and enjoying the fun part of getting to know the new baby's personality and habits, you realize that there is no turning back. So I started to write my birth plan. This time, instead of naively asking for what I wanted, I phrased it as "I Do NOT Need." I had a whole list: I do not need drugs, I do not need surgery, I do not need a hospital gown, I do not need an audience, I do not need negative comments or coercion, etc. It made me feel strong and confident.

I had read a lot about birth on the Internet this time and I found alternative information about natural birth. My favorite imagery was about how you don't need to push; you just let the river flow. I learned about how your uterus changes from contractions that pull the cervix open, to pushing the baby down and out. The trend to be coached or coerced to hold your breath and "purple push" is not how it has to be. I also read about "free birthing" where you just have a private birth and catch your own baby. I liked the idea of just letting the baby be born peacefully at home. We didn't know any home birth midwives in our area, and since our state government did not support them, they couldn't exactly advertise. I'd read an article in a newspaper about women renting houses across the border in the next state. We couldn't really see that working with two little ones, and it still wouldn't be *home* anyway.

I tried to picture the room at our hospital birth center as a rental space where I could birth the way that I needed. The children could stay home in their own space, and I could focus on the birth without worrying about them too. But I told my husband that if they threatened me or upset me in any way that I would leave, and he would have to drive me. I had a back-up plan of renting a hotel room across the street, and I could use the tub and eat whatever I wanted. But our favorite fantasy was calling the midwife from our practice that actually lives one mile from our home and having her come over to our house instead of us all driving 45 minutes away.

I loved the idea of having the baby at home, but I couldn't actually figure out how that would work with 2-year-olds to care for. I tried to picture myself laboring quietly and peacefully somewhere at home, but I don't have any space like that. If I sat down, they were in my lap. They followed me into the bathroom. They slept in my arms. So, they were a big part of this new birth plan. My sister was living with us, and she was nice enough to offer to take time off from work if needed, so she could stay with them, and we could just leave whenever we needed to go, and they would be in their own home with someone that they knew and loved. I made a little poem for her to read to them about the special day, and about becoming a big brother and a big sister. I also bought them supplies so that they could keep busy preparing a "birth"-day party while I was away.

By 37 weeks I was ready for the baby to be born. During the hot summer days, my husband would often play with the kids while I read in the hammock. It was a wonderful summer, but it kept getting hotter and we had visited every friend who had a pool and I would float in the nearby lakes while the kids played in the sand. Since everyone needs to coordinate their schedules so far in advance, my family had made vacation plans before they knew that I was pregnant. The week of my due date we had family coming in to town and had a campsite reserved over at the lake. We would have postponed, but my older brother announced that he was moving away, and everyone wanted one last family get-together. I protested, since I wanted to focus on the birth, but they said that they would help with the kids so that I could relax. We would stay in town and sleep at home at night and only hang out at the campsite during the days if it was nice weather.

So, my parents and brothers came to stay in my house when I was 40 weeks pregnant. I typed up a list of fun places that they could take the kids, complete with directions. The kids could have fun day trips and I could relax at home, take a bath, and maybe go into labor. It sounded like a great plan. You'd think that I would have learned after all these years, that I take care of them; they do not take care of me. I am the one who gets everything planned, then gets everyone up and moving, and constantly tries to make sure that everyone's needs are met. I take care of all the little details that try to keep the peace. But they promised that this time it would be different, and I wanted so badly to believe them. But I guess old habits die hard. Every morning I would try to suggest one of the places on the list while I got breakfast ready and the kids dressed and ready for the day, but no one budged. Now my mom was reading in my hammock instead of me, and my brothers were parked on my couch, and I had more people to cook for and to clean up after.

Each night I would have some time to myself and I would have some good contractions every few minutes, but then they would spread out again as soon as I was focused on meeting everyone else's needs. To make matters worse, that week my mother's depression was worse than ever. I didn't know what to do. She didn't even seem like herself. Her body was here, but it seemed empty, like whatever was really her was completely gone. I held it together through the day, but then when night came I shook and cried because I needed my mother and she was, in essence, gone. I had to mourn that loss and then let that go with big sobs before I could even consider giving birth. I had pictured having my family surrounding me with love and support, but their visit ended up being just one more obstacle. At my 42-week appointment I was so focused on my family that I had no energy for birth.

We still had the reservations at the campsite, so my husband and I took the kids and went to the lake. I tried to just get up and leave without worrying about what everyone else was going to do for the day, but I couldn't do it. I broke down and told my parents and my siblings where we were going, and they showed up at the beach but they hadn't packed any snacks or lunches for themselves, so we cut our sandwiches in half and shared. We spent the day swimming and canoeing and the kids loved digging in the sand. I was hoping to have my family take care of me or help with the kids, but I felt like I was entertaining guests. I guess my family eventually noticed that I wasn't planning to cook anything for them, so they gave up and went out to dinner. But they didn't offer to bring back anything for us. My husband and I stayed and let the kids keep playing in the sand. I walked along the beach and talked to the baby in my belly. The lake and the moonlight were so soothing and calming. As I focused on the baby and the birth, the contractions came stronger and stronger.

Since the lake was an hour-and-a-half away from the hospital, we put the kids in the car and drove back to our house so we could get them settled in their beds and be closer to the birth center since it seemed like things were finally moving along. But when I walked into my house and immediately saw the piles of dirty laundry that my brothers had left on the living room floor, I was so mad that the contractions just stopped completely. When I saw the midwife at my appointment on Monday afternoon, she stripped my membranes to "get things going" a little stronger. I got really crampy, but I am not sure if that's what worked, or if it was that my family finally left. An hour after my last brother drove away, the contractions changed. My husband and my sister and the babies were all asleep and I was up cleaning the house. With my home quiet and returning to order, I could finally breathe. I was standing in the kitchen when I got a contraction so strong that I grabbed the counter and had to stop what I was doing. Instead of big muscular contractions in my belly, I was getting strong pains down my back and in the lower part of my uterus. They kept coming like that for a few hours while I finished everything on my mental to-do list. I woke up my sister and asked her to sleep on the futon in the kids' room so that she would be there when they woke up. Then I woke up my husband and told him that it was time. "Time for what?" he said.

So, we had a nice 45-minute drive down the highway in the middle of the night with the road all to ourselves. After a few attempts to park the car, which is apparently much harder when he is tired and anxious, he took off towards the entrance to the birth center. Too bad I was still leaning on the car finishing a contraction. He looked kind of funny, but the man at the door was sympathetic to the plight of the nervous dad. Finally, we both got settled into the spacious room with the shiny wood floors and equipment on the walls, reminiscent of gym class. After they were done bothering me with multiple attempts at inserting a saline lock for a potential IV, they left us alone. We were back in the same college town where we had met years before, and we were looking out the window at the familiar view, and we were finally ready. We danced in the moonlight and had a nice night together. Since having the babies we had not spent a night alone together slow dancing, so we appreciated stopping everything for a moment and just looking into each other's eyes.

It wasn't all fun and games though. The nurse came to check on me, and asked me to lay on the bed so that she could run a strip on the electronic fetal monitor. I tried to comply, but I could not lie on my back at all. I got up and leaned on the side of the bed. When the midwife came she said "oh, I see you are having some back labor." That was all. No explanation of what that meant or what to do about it to make it better. I have had back pain in my lumbar region from scoliosis since I was a kid, and I had been seeing a chiropractor for years. But having a skull push against that exact spot was excruciating. It was amazing though how manageable labor was without Pitocin. On Pitocin, the contraction peaks and then comes down a little, but the pain never really goes away. Now I was working hard through the contraction and the pain would burn in my spine, but then it would go away entirely in between. I'd pause and squat, holding on to the ballet bar on the wall, and I'd concentrate on my counted breathing. Then, when it was over, I'd hop back on the birth ball and go back to talking and joking with my husband.

When I thought the pain in my back would burn

through me, my husband was there to put counter-pressure on that spot with one hand, and hold me in the other arm. And when another nurse came to "run a strip", the first nurse told her that I couldn't do it, and they didn't try to force me onto my back. The midwife found a way to monitor the baby without disturbing me. I never felt like I needed to run away from the staff. My midwife was done with her shift, but the day before when she stripped my membranes she had promised to stay with me if I came in that night. Labor kept progressing and I knew that I was doing it.

Then transition hit. I knew it felt different and when I saw them wheel in a shiny tray full of stainless steel instruments I was excited to think that I would be done soon. Afterward, my husband told me that he was terrified when they brought in the tools. But mostly what I noticed was that I was now removed from the whole thing, as if I was watching myself. The joking was over. No more looking out the window romantically. No more making funny helicopter sounds by moving the birth ball in a circular motion with my hips. Now it was serious, like a prayer, and I went somewhere deep inside myself.

They moved me to the shower to spray warm water on my back. The water felt nice, but they had taken my clothes and I just couldn't relax standing there naked in the shower with an audience. Then I felt like I needed to poop. The midwife said it was the baby's head pushing on my rectum and it was okay, but I figured the best thing was to be on the toilet, just in case. At least I could relax those perineal muscles there. There was a midwife there with me, and she held my knees tenderly and told me that I could stay there if I wanted, but if the baby came she'd ask me to scoot forward a little so she could catch them. I remember thinking that it was great that she was so caring and accommodating, but who was she? I'd never met this midwife before, and was wondering why she was even here squatting between my legs when my own midwife had promised to stay with me.

My legs were falling asleep from sitting on the toilet for so long, so I moved to the bed. I leaned on some pillows on the back of the bed while I kneeled. It felt so comfortable and I'd been up all night, so I went to sleep. I woke up with each contraction, but they felt different. It felt like my uterus was pushing the baby down. I kept thinking, "let the river flow; don't push it." I slept like that for over an hour, waking with each contraction and kind of observing it, but totally detached. I had my back to the room and was focusing on the wall outlets. My husband was by my side. The midwife was there the whole time, rubbing oil on my perineum and waiting.

When my knees gave out, the midwife suggested that I move to a semi-sitting position. When I turned, I saw that my midwife had come back, but was standing there wearing street clothes and watching me while the stranger was between my legs. With each contraction the baby came down but then slipped back again. It was frustrating, but just when I was getting worried the midwife explained that it is exactly what is supposed to happen. After my uterus had been pushing the baby down for 2 hours, the head was crowning, and the midwife said that I would actually have to give a push now. I would get to the point where the head was stretching the tissue and I felt that "ring of fire", and then I would retreat. I needed to force myself to push past that. I gave myself a little pep talk in my head, telling myself to just push out the head, and then I'd worry about the shoulders and the rest of the body later. So, with the next contraction I gritted my teeth and pushed past the burning. With that, the head came flying out, followed by the whole body and before I could breathe there was a new baby lying on my chest.

I looked quickly and I saw something between the legs, but then I realized that it was the umbilical cord. There was something else there too though, and just as I had suspected, it was a brand new baby boy. He latched right on to my breast and started nursing and they said that by about 2 hours they would want to take him for his measurements etc. We were back to joking and talking while they sewed a single stitch for a small tear which the midwife said wasn't too bad for a baby being born backwards with a raised fist presenting along with his head. I was back to being a breastfeeding mom and it felt wonderful. But this time I was a beautiful, strong and proud VBAC mom.

He had been born in the middle of the morning, and after the two hours of bonding and snuggling, I was ready to get up and go pee and get dressed in something pretty. My husband took the baby over to the bassinet to get weighed and measured. I called home and talked to my sister and then told my kids that they had a baby brother. They were excited and they had been keeping busy making cupcakes and decorating the house while they waited. When my husband went to get them later that afternoon, the nurse told me that when they walked through the door they would seem huge. She was right. The day before they had been tiny toddlers; but next to the newborn they were suddenly enormous. I snuggled in the bed with my 3 babies, and I felt true joy.

That night, my husband went home to stay with the twins and left me to rest with the new baby. But I couldn't sleep. I was so high on the birth hormones and endorphins. The baby was too. He was alert and playful and flirting with the nurses. We ended up having a fun girl's-night in my room with a couple of the nurses. Despite working in Labor and Delivery, the nurses didn't often see completely natural birth, and they were amazed that they baby could push with his feet and almost stand up to lunge for the breast when he wanted to nurse. I found it unbelievable that I was telling *them* about birth when they see it every day, and it was really my first time. I talked a mile a minute as I told them about how I had done it, how I had pushed out my baby. I called all my girlfriends and told them they had to try this. This natural high was the best thing I'd ever felt.

I had needed that night to myself in the hospital before going home and having to figure out how to sleep with 3 babies in our bed. But there was still plenty of mommy for everyone. I could sleep with the baby on my chest and one toddler on each side. The days were similar. I just put the baby in the sling and still had one hand free for each of the twins. When they were really tired, I could carry one on each hip. They are not kidding when they say that mothers are strong women. We need to be strong in more ways than our children will ever know.

Chapter 5: Mothering the Mother

Much to my surprise, having a new baby was the easy part of being a mother of three. My children loved the new baby, and if you are diapering two, you might as well diaper three. The four of us kept busy by going to meetings and playgrounds and to playgroups at the library. I could nurse the baby in the sling while I chased after my adventuresome toddlers. He was an easy baby. He never spit up and he never needed to be burped. His needs were simple and I knew how to meet them. Coping with the changing and challenging behaviors of the 2-year-olds was another matter, especially given that they were two totally independent and opposite children. Becoming a mother is hard enough in the first place, but then with each new challenge, you need to become a new kind of mother.

As one challenging day ran into the next, I kept telling myself that everything was fine. Winter came, and it was a cold one. It wasn't just snow; it was ice and bitter cold wind so we ended up being stuck indoors most of the time. I kept feeling like I was slipping away and losing control. I finally turned to the women in my La Leche League group and confided that I may be having some postpartum depression. I had read that it can begin when your monthly cycles return (which mine did at 6 months postpartum this time) and I am sure the dark and cold season didn't help either. It was very hard for me to turn to the group and ask for help, since I had been volunteering as the group leader for a few years and facilitating the meetings. At this point though, I was desperate and I knew I needed support. I felt like I could trust these women.

My personal crisis came at a bad time though since the group chose that winter to reassess the group and propose changes. I had given so much of myself to support the moms in my community and help provide a safe place for them to share and to seek support. But right when I reached out and asked for support from the group, they chose that time to go behind my back and decide on a new way to run the meetings. I was informed in a mean-spirited phone call that my volunteer efforts had not been appreciated, and a few other women felt that they should take over the group instead. I had encouraged mothers from the group to take on different group jobs, but they would not show up to meetings, and not do what they had offered. I would totally understand how hard it is to balance the needs of the group with the needs of your own family so I couldn't blame them. But then I had to cover for them and juggle all of the group jobs myself while caring for my three little ones. I was already hurting and feeling betrayed, when I received that phone call in which one of the women said that she had stopped coming and helping because she "didn't like me." I couldn't imagine saying that to *anyone*, but that is just me I guess. So, these were the women with whom I had been trying to develop friendships. This was my support group. I had thought that they were my friends. Needless to say, this development did not help the postpartum depression.

After that phone call, I felt empty and worthless. I stopped trying to fight the depression. I had tried to be the perfect mother. I had tried to make friends. I had tried to be there for others, and assumed that they would be there for me when I needed them. The next day while the kids played, I just lay on the floor of the play room and sobbed uncontrollably. The kids looked concerned as I shook and big tears splashed onto the floor. I didn't know how to make it stop. I crawled to the phone and I called the church. I was desperately calling for help and I got connected to a secretary who took a message. Nobody ever called me back.

I became obsessed with starting over. I made

elaborate plans to sell everything and move to the other side of the planet. My brother had moved to the other side of planet and when my sister returned from a visit she made it sound like the best place in the world. I wanted to go somewhere that I wouldn't have to fight all the time. I'd find a place where the midwifery model of care is the norm and women can breastfeed in public without judgment. I dreamed of a place where strong, intelligent women are respected and encouraged. There were other countries with better public policies, but they had their own problems too. No place is perfect. Our families were here; our certifications and licenses were all from this state. We had a mortgage on a house that would never sell in this market even if I could imagine leaving it. It would be too hard to start over at this point, the plan was too hard to enact and nothing changed.

During this time, I reached out but couldn't get any emotional support from my mother. When I told her how I was feeling, she just talked about how she had "real" depression and how what I had was basically nothing. I know now that it is probably just that she didn't want me to suffer the way that she had, and maybe she was trying to say that it would get better, but at the time I just needed her to hear me. I had been having episodes of depression for years and had developed my own strategies to deal with it, and had never had to use prescription medication. This time though, with the hormones and the dramatic change to my routine and my whole identity as a person, the depression brought me deeper than ever and I had no idea where to turn. As a mother myself now, it was easy to understand how the postpartum depression had affected my mother so strongly. But she had always tried really hard to keep functioning because being a good mom was so important to her. It wasn't until my sister went into the hospital for brain surgery that she really was brought to a point where she didn't know how to come back. I lived in constant fear that something would happen that would push me over that edge.

Since I was a little girl I had told everyone that I wanted to be a mom and to have a family. I had gone all the way through graduate school and was really interested in my field, but even more important than any degrees or titles, I studied because I really wanted to understand health and I taught because I wanted to share what I had learned with others. Now that I was a mom, I didn't want to miss these years with my children. I had originally planned to be home with my babies when they were small, but by the time I actually had kids I was so used to the status of my career. It defined who I was, and now that was gone. I had thrown myself into volunteer positions and did the hard work of getting accredited as a La Leche League Leader in order to support other new moms, but also because I needed to have a larger purpose. All of the reading and studying and running the group had kept me intellectually stimulated and focused. Now that was gone too.

I think a huge part of the postpartum depression and my inability to "snap out of it" came from not knowing who I was, or where to go next. In this culture, your identity is so wrapped up in what you do for a living. After my first pregnancy I was just out on maternity leave. This time though, I knew that I wasn't going back to my job. I had devoted 7 years of higher education, and then 5 more years to get my program just the way I wanted it, and now I had to leave that behind. I couldn't keep commuting so far and working so many hours and be the kind of mom that I had wanted to be.

During this time I felt like the weight of the world was on my shoulders. I couldn't make a decision about anything because I would think of all of the possible ramifications of that choice. I couldn't buy anything at the store because the amount of choices and the consequences were crippling. What if I bought something and then it was recalled and I had put the children in danger? What if that chemical they claim is safe turns out to have negative effects once they do further studies years from now? What if the factory it was made in uses child labor? Does that company have unfair labor practices? If I stayed home I'd go stir-crazy, but if I left the house I had to use gasoline to get to town and then I'd feel guilty about the soldiers that were dying in the wars over petroleum. And then at the playground or the library the other mothers would question all of my choices and I didn't have enough answers. I had been brought up to always have an answer, or to do more research, more homework. I felt so unprepared for this job of motherhood, and it was so overwhelming.

I found a therapist who specializes in postpartum depression. I thought it would be great, she would tell me what to do. She gave me solutions that she said were easy, like that I should just meditate. But meditation did not seem easy, it felt impossible. I couldn't turn off these negative thoughts, and sitting with them longer didn't seem constructive. She told me not to worry about the babies in Africa or the migrant workers, but how could I stop? She told me to exercise, and I tried, but I couldn't carve out a minute to myself. Doing yoga with someone climbing on you is hard. You can go for a walk but your demons go with you. Sitting quietly and meditating with the chaos all around me was even harder. I needed time, but I was afraid to take it, and I was afraid to be alone with my thoughts.

I did finally pick up the phone and talk to my aunt, and it was really hard to do because I felt like I was admitting defeat. Actually, it turned out to be just what I needed. She told me stories about how she was losing her mind and going a little crazy when she was home with small children. Her confession made me feel like I was not alone, and reassured me to no end because she had always represented my image of a good mother. She sent me the book *Gift From the Sea* by Anne Morrow Lindbergh in the mail, and opening that package was the beginning of a turning point (4). It is a short, almost poetic book, and an easy read even with babies to care for all hours of the day. But the book is profound in its simplicity, like the seashells she respects and admires. In reading this book I finally felt like someone understood. There are so many things that I want to accomplish in this world and in this lifetime, but first I need to be at peace with myself. Maybe this time in my life was an opportunity to slow down and reflect, and start over in a way.

In more ways than one, this book was a godsend. In this book I found the understanding that I hadn't gotten from the therapist. I felt like she was downplaying the importance of all these huge decisions that were consuming my mind and my existence. In this book though, Mrs. Lindbergh describes similar thoughts. She speaks of the fact that our society is so large that our efforts and our womanly acts of giving of ourselves can get lost in the sheer distance. It is our instinct to give and to nurture, but in this ever-growing global community there are too many needs to fill. "We are linked to more people than our hearts can hold."(4) We drain ourselves and need to find ways to refill the pitcher. So, maybe the therapist was right about the meditation, but first I needed to hear that someone understood my concerns, and that they were valid. Not only did this author understand, but my aunt must have understood since she knew this book was exactly what I needed. Now, instead of feeling like something was wrong with me, I could feel like I was a part of a larger sisterhood of caring women.

In this book about the sea, she describes how each shell is "fitted and formed by its own life and struggle to survive."(4) After having a baby, you look down one day and realize that you don't even recognize this body that you inhabit. I had always felt like my true self, my spiritual being, was separate from the body that I was given for this life. But now I kind of missed my body. One day the kids were being impossible, and I cried in the shower when I saw the body that I had ruined, for them. I could never go back to looking like a young woman again. I would think of those crime shows where they can tell all the details about the person when they find the body, and I would think that with all these stretch marks and scars there was no question that I had children. I would get envious of my husband who could go out and take a break and pretend that he had no children if he wanted. He could go back to being his old self, and no one would ever know that he was a father. He looked exactly the same as before. I had stretch marks from my shoulders to my knees. But while I read *A Gift from the Sea*, I could finally start to appreciate the fact that my shell held the marks of my accomplishments. (4)

I needed to appreciate the "ebb and flow of life," for "each cycle of the tide is valid."(4) In this book she emphasizes that we need to find simplicity, integrity and fuller relationships. If we only always make friends with people who are like ourselves, we will never grow. We need to make the effort to understand others who are different from ourselves. And in making the effort, we learn more about our true selves. After each change, it takes time to come to terms with yourself in your new role, in this new stage of life. I wanted to take this time to find my center and rejuvenate myself and really think about what to do next.

I had waited so long to become a mother, and it was so wonderful to finally be in that stage of my life, at first.

But then it sinks in that there is no going back. I tried to go back to my job, but I couldn't focus on it with the same energy as I had before I was a mom. When my third came along I knew that I needed to make the choice to stay home with them for many reasons. But there is a huge difference between being home on leave for a set period of time, and being home with no job to go back to, and no plan for what to do next. My job hadn't made financial sense anymore with the costs of daycare and gas for the commute. But the savings wouldn't last forever, so I couldn't really relax knowing that I wasn't bringing in any more money.

A few months earlier, I had been so excited about helping the mothers and babies in my community that I had signed up for a doula-training workshop. I thought that providing birth support would be a great way for me to combine my educational and health science background with my new experiences of helping mothers. I would be able to educate them during the prenatal phase, be there to support them during their birth, and then be a resource and source of support after they brought the baby home. I would be able to use my skills and my intellect, and make my own appointments while making some money. I wouldn't be able to make a full salary, but maybe I could at least contribute, and the savings would last a little longer.

At this point though, after all that had happened in my La Leche League group, I was so betrayed and hurt that I couldn't picture being in a room full of women. I couldn't become a part of a group and put myself out there to be rejected again. I figured it was best to just call and cancel my reservation for the workshop. Who would want me to be their doula anyway? It had been a silly idea. I should just stay home. It would be too difficult to leave the children for the weekend, and then I would still have to work to complete my certification. It would be easier to quit now. But I had already done all the reading assignments and loved everything that I read. And besides, maybe a challenge was exactly what I needed.

The depression almost won, and I almost stayed home to wallow in my own self-pity, but in the end I did go to the doula-training workshop. Luckily my husband finally convinced me to go, since the workshop ended up being a real turning point for me It was the first time I had left my twins overnight, except for when I gave birth to their brother, but it was local so I could come home if I was needed. My in-laws came to help keep them entertained and to help my husband for the long weekend. The baby was only 7 months old, so he wasn't moving around too much yet, and was used to going everywhere in the sling and nursing night and day, so he went with me. I'm really glad that I made it there, since that weekend changed my life.

I had my reservations about meeting new people at this point, and I figured I would just go and focus on learning the content, and not to make friends. But the women I met that weekend were the most "real" women I had ever met. In between the sessions, it was not just time passed in small talk, it was real and deep discussion. There were women there from diverse backgrounds and they had all different styles and personalities. Each one of these women brought something unique to the group, but what they had in common was that they all seemed truly open and caring.

One thing that really amazed me that weekend was the way some of these women viewed health in a totally different way than what I was raised to believe. I had used the definition in graduate school that health is "not merely the absence of disease, but a state of physical, emotional, and spiritual well-being." But despite agreeing with that statement in principle, I lived in a culture where we just list all the things that are wrong, then treat the symptoms, or use drugs to make sure we don't feel anything. This was the first time that I met people who actually believed that being truly healthy was really an option.

They even encouraged us to really pay attention to

the language that we use in our culture. It is amazing how much power there is in the way that you describe something. I began to notice more about how negative women in this culture are about their bodies and their health. Just by choosing positive language I could start to change my belief structure. It is like when they say that you can feel better just by smiling, even if it is not spontaneous and you have to force yourself to change your expression; just the mere act of smiling changes how you feel. I needed to really believe that true health was attainable before I could begin to heal.

Just as an example, think about all the ways in which women can describe their menstruation. There is that term: menstruation (which we all learned in health class) but nobody uses that in conversation. I've heard that you are "getting a monthly gift," or that "Aunt Flo is visiting" from people trying to be delicate. Usually teenage boys describe it more crudely with expressions like "on the rag," or "riding the crimson wave." Men also refer to the "women's curse." Most women I knew just tried to avoid talking about it if at all possible. In my family it was called your "period," but it was better if it was not mentioned at all. My grandmother never even talked to my mother about it once. Imagine her surprise the first time. How refreshing to hear women just matter-of-factly talk about when they are "bleeding." They just come right out and state the facts like there is nothing wrong with it and there is no reason to be ashamed. They would also refer to their "cycles," acknowledging that there is a rhythm and a purpose and all is at it should be.

There are also so many ways to refer to the "private" parts of our own bodies. Just starting with that term, "private parts" sets the theme for how we treat certain parts of our bodies in this culture. From the time we are small, we learn when we can show these parts, and to whom. Many of us learn to hate these parts of our bodies, and become ashamed of them. That weekend there were women who spoke of their sacred spot, or their yoni. Although I never spoke about mine, I had never heard it called anything but a "vagina." I was shocked when I found out that "vagina" means "sheath for a sword," referring to its role in sex. After that, when speaking about birth, I would only call it the Birth Canal, since it is now a passageway for a baby. You can also use the proper term "vulva" referring to the external female genitalia (now there is a good textbook word for you). I remember being on the playground as a young girl and being told, "boys have a penis, girls have a vagina." Instead of referring to the vulva or the labia that they know are there because they are external, they use the word vagina referring to a part of their body that they probably haven't even discovered yet. So, from a very young age, girls are defining their bodies in terms of how they will be used by someone else. And the medical model and most of the textbooks these girls will ever see refer to women's bodies in how they are different from the male counterpart. A male body in this culture is considered normal and healthy, and so women by definition must be wrong, unhealthy, and even cursed.

With this realization, I knew that I wanted to do whatever I could to raise my daughter with some self-esteem, despite our cultural views of women. When I went home from the workshop, I would try to use positive language about her body, and my own, too. Since she was still potty training, we had plenty of opportunities to discuss that part of the body. I would talk with her about keeping that part of her body clean, and we'd talk about how she has a special hole where babies come out. At her age she doesn't need to think about sex, and I don't want her own body to be defined in terms of some future man's. I want her to grow up being proud of her body, not ashamed. But I was raised to be proper, and I want her to respect herself, so I encourage her to dress properly so that when the time comes, it is up to her when and how people see her or touch her there. I also know what kind of culture we live in and I want her to be safe. We talk about the importance of keeping that area covered to stay clean and healthy, but not because it is of itself "dirty" and needs to be hidden.

So, in the same vein, at this doula-training workshop we learned how to use better language when speaking to other women about birth. Instead of saying that her "water broke," you can say that her "waters released," which is technically more accurate and also removes the negative imagery. In movies and on television about 100% of the women have their water break in some dramatic way, usually in a huge gush, in public, with no warning, leaving a huge puddle behind as they rush to the hospital in full on labor. So, in real life, when it is your first pregnancy, you wait for your dramatic scene. You wonder where and when it will happen to you. But if in real life, you are one of the 80-90% of women who enter active labor with your membranes intact, you feel like something must be wrong with you.

In addition to the positive terminology to use in conversation, there is also the textbook term which is "spontaneous rupture of membranes" or SROM. Now that sounds dramatic enough to fit in with the Hollywood scenes a little more, but the percentages are way off. And even when the waters release, it could be just a trickle or a slow leak where you are left wondering if you just wet yourself. Very few women actually have a huge gush of fluids. By the time you are full term with a baby's head pushing right on your bladder, that seems totally feasible that you would be leaking urine. Luckily there is a litmus test to tell you which is going on, because when your life is not summed up into a 2-hour movie or a half hour sitcom, it is not so easy to figure out.

Of course, if all that describes the spontaneous rupture that happens to about 20% of the women in the real world, what about the rest of us? If you arrive at the hospital in active labor, or stalled labor, or potential labor, they may want to "just break your water", to "get things moving." They say it as if it is nothing, and you consent because you are already wondering what is wrong with you that you missed your dramatic entrance. So, here they come to perform what is called an "artificial rupture of membranes" or AROM, further establishing who is the boss of your body. If they used the proper term and asked if they could "artificially rupture your membranes," you might actually stop to think about the procedure they are about to perform. You might even want to ask about the potential implications, side effects, or complications of the procedure. But why offer the woman the opportunity for informed consent, when she might say "no." It is easier for the staff if everyone just pretends that it is no big deal.

There is a lot of power in the language that we choose. If we start to choose positive language about birth, then maybe we can start to glimpse some of the beauty and the magic that there is in it. Maybe we will find that our bodies are healthy and strong. Blessed, not cursed. Just having that realization opened a door for me that I never even knew was there, like when Mary finds the door to the secret garden.

Chapter 6: Opening Up to More

I had a lot of "aha" moments the weekend of the birth doula training. A lot of the things I learned I probably already knew in a way, but never realized because they were so far outside of my belief structure. Another thing that was new for me that weekend was how the doulas in the group spoke about energy. Not just in terms of having "enough" energy, but in having the right kind of energy, like how we each bring a different kind of energy to each relationship and each experience. We learned about bringing positive energy to the birth. If labor wasn't progressing, maybe you needed to change the energy. Many of the things we learned were quite intuitive, but just the fact that they were covered in the curriculum at all really challenged the way that I saw the world.

I come from a family that values science and logic. Every time I make a statement about anything, I need to back it up with evidence or data. I could never say that I "just knew it". To truly trust your intuition, you need to be okay with tuning in to your body, and trusting that it will tell you when the energy is not right. And it was exactly that type of thing that I really needed to learn more about in order to become a doula. How could I ask another woman to trust me, when I did not trust myself? How could I ask her to listen to her body, when I did not listen to mine? It became clear that my problem was not in trusting birth. I had read all the statistics and I knew that natural birth was possible. I knew logically that it was safe and healthy. But as soon as I was thrown into the challenge of actually facing birth head on, I reverted to that belief structure that was ingrained in me since childhood, and I assumed that there was something wrong with me. After all, my body hated me, and I hated my body.

To truly be there to support other women, I needed to be strong myself. To be able to reach out to others, I needed to first be able to trust my own body. I needed to love myself. I had been suffering from low self-esteem my whole life, so this was not going to be easy. I had been to all kinds of specialists and had exploratory surgeries, but no doctor had ever found anything medically wrong with me, and yet I kept having symptoms. In reality, my own language was pointing to the answer all along. Since I had no medical diagnosis, if people asked me what I had, I would just say, "Oh, my body hates me." I had this person that I felt was my true self, and then there was this body that could be hurt and used; the body that had often betrayed me. Could it be that this body that I was so ashamed of had in fact been trying to tell me something? I had always felt like my *self* and my *body* were two totally separate things. There is no wonder that birth, where your rational brain shuts off, and you need to be present in your body, had been so difficult for me.

I did learn a lot of the science of birth that weekend. I learned positions and techniques and hands-on skills. But what I really learned from those women shook me to my core. Something was awakened inside of me. When we were sent forth from the training, we were encouraged to go and do whatever it was that we needed to do in order to be truly ready, before we began our work as doulas. For the first time in my life, I really felt like I *could* be healed, and I felt like I needed it, but more importantly I felt like I *deserved* it.

It is amazing to me how I can be completely blind to things that are right in front of me because I do not allow myself to see them. And sometimes, the exact thing that I didn't even know I needed is put right in my path, precisely when I need it. One way in which it always catches my attention is at the bookstore. You can walk through there every day and depending on what is going on in your life, you will be drawn to different titles or designs. I always seem to find exactly what I need, even if I didn't know what I was seeking. Once in college, I was drawn to a bright orange book and when I picked it up and leafed through it randomly, the paragraph I read was about my cousin. This book included the story of when she had died suddenly of a mystery virus and even mentioned her by name. I walked in a trance to the cash register and handed it to the cashier with shaking hands. When I got home and read through the whole book it confirmed why I had chosen that career path in the first place. The next semester it was required reading for my "Plagues, Politics and People" class.

This time as I walked through my favorite bookstore, fresh from my doula training, and seeing the world through new eyes, I wandered into a new section and looked right at a title that had been mentioned at the training. It was a used book store, so the inventory is kind of hit or miss, so the fact that there was a copy of *Women's Bodies, Women's Wisdom: Creating Physical and Emotional Health and Healing* by Christiane Northrup, MD waiting there just for me might have been more than just coincidence (5). Books, like friends, seem to come into my life right when I need them. Anyway, this book was over 600-pages long, and despite the fact that I had three little ones, I managed to read it cover to cover. It did take a while, but not just because of the kids. I had to stop and take notes because there were so many profound passages that I needed to be able to come back to and process further.

Women's Bodies, Women's Wisdom introduced me to the idea of "healing verses curing" and "listening to your body", but the section where she really grabbed my attention was when she reviewed the concept of chakras. (5) These are ancient principles, but she wrote about them in an approachable context. There are seven energy centers in our bodies that are affected by emotional and psychological issues and can manifest in physical symptoms. As I read through her examples, I was shocked to find explanations for my medical symptoms that had as yet stumped every physician and every test they could give me. For each of the things that had caused me to visit doctors over the years, there were really profound links to what was going on in my life at the time the symptoms started.

When I was in third grade, they had a police officer come to our class to talk to us about speaking out if someone made you do something that you didn't want to do with your body. They said that we were supposed to tell, and that they would take care of us, and we wouldn't get in trouble. They asked if any of us wanted to talk to the officer, and when I raised my hand I was taken out into the hall. I told him about how my teenaged neighbor would make me pull down my pants so he could look at my private parts. (Not that he was the only one, but he was a bully so I didn't feel like I needed to protect him. I think it was also a cry for help that I hoped would open up a chance for me to talk about the other things that were bothering me.) I had felt so dirty and ashamed, that I had never told. Now they made me feel like a good girl for telling the truth, and they had promised that I would be protected.

When the police came to my neighborhood that afternoon to question my neighbors, they were less than pleased to have someone prying. Apparently, seeing the police come to the neighborhood upset one of the neighbors. She was running her home-based business off the books, and was always nervous about being caught. When they found out why the police were there, I was punished for speaking out and making the neighbors worry. My parents were embarrassed that I now had a case on file with child protective services. I was so shocked that this whole thing had backfired. They did not protect me as promised. Nothing was said about the neighbor who had done it. They continued to live next door, and nothing changed. I was already carrying too many secrets and I had thought that this would be a way to start getting some help. Instead, I learned not to trust adults, not to trust the police or my teachers, and not to tell the truth. I internalized the message that "nobody likes a tattle-tale." And I learned to never ask for help.

By fourth grade I had developed a blocked salivary gland that would swell until it burst open in my mouth, leaving me unable to speak until I found something to spit it all into. They tried to remove the blockage surgically, but it grew back. I was taken to more specialists, who had never seen anything like it, so they cut out the whole gland. Then I grew a tumor on my neck. In Dr. Northrup's book, she describes the 5th chakra in the mouth and throat as being affected by issues with personal expression. Physical symptoms in that area arise when you cannot use your personal power. Not being able to speak up or stand up for yourself can also affect your vertebrae and cause scoliosis. I failed that screening test in 5th grade. After reading this book and making that connection, I tried to talk about the whole incident with my mother. She told me that I had been mistaken and completely denied that there was even an older boy living in that house when I was growing up. Just in case I was actually going crazy, I called my older brother to confirm that the neighbor did in fact exist. My mother uses amazing amounts of denial as her coping strategy for just about everything.

So, there were two medical mysteries solved after all these years of specialists, tests, surgeries and procedures. But how do you explain my "episodes?" What was causing those debilitating pains that was so elusive to medical science? Why wasn't it cured by bland diets, or pharmaceuticals, or chiropractic? It is very easy to become frustrated by a health care system that has no answers and doesn't take care of us, or promote health.

Reading *Women's Bodies, Women's Wisdom* helped me to understand how my history of being hurt and victimized had been internalized and was causing my physical symptoms. After a childhood in which I had been hurt by neighbors and friends and even family members, a series of physically and emotionally abusive relationships in high school finally pushed me over the edge and I started to have "episodes" of physical pain.

Reading through the descriptions in the book was like an overview of my past experiences, cross-referenced with my medical chart. Asthma is a symptom of the 4th chakra caused by a decrease in love of life or an inability to give love to yourself. Lack of self-esteem, fear, intimidation and the inability to trust others can all manifest in intestinal problems and eating disorders. Blame and guilt, problems with sex and a loss of power and control in the physical world (rape) is all remembered in the lower chakras, the female energy centers. My pelvic pain and low back pain, urinary infections and gynecological problems could all be linked to this. Chronic low back pain and hip pain indicate that you are not able to stand up for yourself, that you are not supported by anyone, and that you do not feel safe in the world. I was on the track team in school, but the hip pain and asthma kept me from winning, but more to the point, it made me feel like I couldn't run away fast enough. I felt stuck in this body that hated me.

I read the rest of that book, and then I went on to read more of the books that Christiane Northrup had mentioned, particularly *Anatomy of the Spirit: The Seven Stages of Power and Healing* by Caroline Myss (6) and *Revolution from Within: A Book of Self-Esteem* by Gloria Steinem (7). Dr. Caroline Myss is a medical intuitive and a practitioner of energy medicine. In her book she shows how you can go through Seven Stages of Spiritual Growth and find your own personal power, and if you do that you can heal your physical body as well. Unlike when we look for a cure to stop the progression of a disease, true healing requires an active internal process in which we release our own negative emotional patterns. She gives examples of how you can really start to recognize how you are using your energy, so that you can then begin to use your energy for the creation of love, self-esteem and consequently, physical and spiritual health. I finally felt like I was on to something, but this entire process of discovery just helped me to realize how much work there was to be done. I had looked into myself and found my wounds, and these books helped to legitimize my pain. Now I really needed to start finding ways to heal.

In her book *Revolution from Within*, Gloria Steinem not only explores the meaning and the importance of self-esteem, she shows you how to nurture it in your own life. One part that really spoke to me was when she describes how you can visualize your future self, and in your meditations, you can picture this stronger, healthier, future self taking care of your inner child, even if your current self cannot. Your future self can be the "mother" that you need, one that truly knows and understands both you and your inner child. We need to navigate the present circumstances of our lives, but we can use the creativity of our inner child, and the wisdom of our future self, to help us to live in this moment. We need to love and care for ourselves, as much as we love and care for others.

In *Anatomy of the Spirit*, Caroline Myss says that the truth is delivered to us through life's challenges, and there is nowhere that I have seen this to be more evident than during a birth. In other aspects of our lives we find that we can delay a challenge, make excuses, or get out of it somehow. When it comes time for a baby to be born, we cannot avoid the challenge. They have tried over many generations to find ways to numb the feelings, or extract the baby surgically, but not without consequences. There are lessons to be learned from the birth, for both the mother and the child, and science is starting to find more and more evidence that if you try to postpone or avoid the physical pain, or even to speed up the process, there will be even greater challenges ahead. It can take up to 2 weeks for the effects of the drugs to wear off in a baby. The baby can be lethargic, fussy, or some may say colicky. Those two weeks are the most critical in the baby's life, a time to initiate breastfeeding, create emotional bonds, and establish other patterns that will be carried out throughout the child's life.

There are numerous books and studies that explain how important the process of labor is for the final stages of development from fetus to infant. If the baby is denied the work of those contractions, then there could be developmental delays. Ashley Montagu presented these phenomena in his book *Touching, The Human Significance of the Skin (8)*. Although he first published this book in 1971, women today still need to ask for their babies to be brought to them right away for skin-to-skin contact and "kangaroo care" is finally being promoted in some NICUs. Reading this book during my first pregnancy had made me aware of the importance of contractions and labor. I told a nurse that even if I needed a cesarean, I still wanted to wait until I'd had some active labor so that the babies would not be deprived of the final stages of development. She thought I was crazy to *want* to labor. As a medical professional working with pregnant and birthing mothers, she had never learned about the importance of labor beyond the uterine contractions pushing the baby down and out. There are many aspects and dimensions of birth that I'm sure are yet to be discovered.

In a natural birth, there is physical pain, and emotional and spiritual challenges, but they are not there without reason. When the doctor or nurse presents you with the question "do you want pain, or no pain?" what do you think you would choose? But it is a misleading question. There isn't an option of "no pain" in life, even with amazing amounts of procrastination or avoidance. Many times a drugged labor means that the mother will need either a surgical birth by cesarean section, or a forceps-assisted birth with an episiotomy. Recovery for the mother is much harder from a surgical birth, or with complications from an epidural or the use of instruments. In those cases, the pain was delayed, but now the mother is home caring for a fussy infant and trying to recover from her own physical and emotional wounds. And they forget to tell you that with a natural labor come these amazing hormones that provide pain-relief ten times stronger than morphine, and without negative side effects.

There are other things that the medical professionals don't want you to know about natural birth. They may want to discuss what your plan is for handling the pain of labor, but they don't tell you that many women have the best emotional and spiritual high of their life, and some even call it orgasmic. If they told you that you were going to have the most amazing experience of your life, and possibly the best orgasm, would you still choose to numb the experience? But in the sterile world of the hospital, it is embarrassing for them to think of women as sensual creatures. They make every effort to make you look and feel just like every other patient. On this most beautiful day when you are bringing forth new life, you are dressed like the old man with cancer on the next floor up.

Even the term "natural birth" has become clouded with confusion over the past few decades. Many people use the term to mean vaginal birth verses a surgical birth. Many women (like me) think that they need to avoid pain-medication, to show that they can handle it. But there is also an increasing trend in hospital births to try to augment, or speed up the labor with artificial hormones. When they use the artificial Pitocin, it shuts down your own body's production of Oxytocin, and then you do not get the natural painkillers, you do not get the natural high or the good feelings. With Pitocin you also do not get any breaks between contractions to rest and recover. Pitocin brings on stronger, more painful and more frequent contractions, which obviously is not great for the mother, and is not so pleasant for the baby either. But they are poised for surgery if there is any sign of distress. And don't worry, they usually start the Pitocin on Monday or Tuesday morning, not on Fridays, so it won't interfere with their plans for the weekend. If you are being difficult, and think of staying pregnant too long, they will find something to make you worry. You may conveniently start to show signs of too much or too little fluid, too high or too low blood pressure, or the baby may be too large. It's like those movies where the scary music starts, and you know something is coming. Even if they tell you everything is totally normal, but they say it in a scary tone, it will give you a sense of foreboding and bring on the stress-response of fight-or-flight and make you feel like you need to *do* something.

The next thing you know, you are in an ugly gown and tied to the IV pole, with little hope of walking or taking a bath or any of the other things you saw on the birth video in childbirth education class. Instead of a gradual labor in which you can learn to handle the contractions, you are thrown into full-speed-ahead labor without warning. At this point, they ask you if you still want to be a martyr, or if you are ready for them to give you an epidural. After all, you are starting to make some noise and be a little annoying to the staff. So, the epidural can give everyone a break. Sounds great, except that you were supposed to be having a baby, and now they've given you a drug that stops labor. But that's okay, more Pitocin is on hand, and if that doesn't work fast enough, they have an operating room all prepped and ready.

After I completed my doula training, I had to take a childbirth education class as part of my certification process. Most of the women in the class were first time mothers, but there was one woman who was pregnant with her second child. She had given birth about seven years before and had been down the roller coaster of interventions. On the first day of class, she was quite abrasive and said that she was just going to have a cesarean to avoid the whole managed labor this time. She was there because her partner was a first time dad, and he knew nothing about birth or babies. But as the weeks progressed, it became more and more clear that she was just scared. As I talked with her more over the breaks and after class, it was clear that in fact, she really wanted a natural labor and birth, but that wasn't what she got the first time and didn't think it was really possible in this hospital. She was also limited by insurance and transportation issues. She thought that she would rather recover from surgery than go through a manipulative and demoralizing labor again.

I offered to work with this couple free of charge, and I started to meet with them in their apartment. When her labor started on Friday night, I drove them to the hospital and they checked her dilation. The labor was going along at a good pace, but then the nurse started asking about her older son. Even though she was clearly upset that she no longer lived with him and rarely saw him, the nurse continued to ask questions. By the time the doctor bothered to pop in to say hello, the labor had just about stopped completely, and I drove them home.

While we had been waiting for the doctor, I had been able to palpate her abdomen and felt that the baby was posterior. I showed her some positions to use to allow the baby to move into an easier position, and then I went home. She had contractions all day Saturday while moving around the apartment on hands-and-knees and her floors got washed and the baby turned to the side. Labor picked up again and I drove them to the hospital in the evening and the doctor checked her progress. She was still in the early stages, but she said that she did not want to use Pitocin because it increases the pain. The doctor was condescending and would not have a discussion with her about medications. My client was put into a position of losing all of her personal power, and the labor stopped.

On Sunday, we checked in to the hospital for good and the labor was pretty steady. I had talked with her about doing what she needed to do, and not worrying about what the nurses or the doctor wanted. She brought her own pretty lamp, and a picture of her son. She wore a really bright tie-dye shirt, a beautiful sarong, and a fluffy bathrobe. I took pictures of her sitting on the birth ball and smiling. We walked the halls again and again while her partner took a nap, and then while he went home for a lunch-break with a shower and a change of clothes. Each time he took a break and left her side, her labor slowed, but it did not stop. I tried to tell him that he was going to be a dad and that there were no breaks, but he said he had to go. He did not understand how much she waited for him. As we walked, she told me her stories. I had the impression that she had a past full of abuse and low self-esteem, and there was nothing really surprising in the stories that she shared, but she needed to tell them. When the baby's head pressed on one side, we put that leg up on the bench in the hall to open that hip. She kept laboring despite the looks from the nurses. Eventually the partner returned, and the labor sped up considerably, and we settled into the room.

Her partner held her and I took pictures of the two of them. She looked at him with such love in her eyes. When she was tired, I gave her a back massage and he rubbed her feet. I think she needed a day of friendship and love and pampering. Then all of a sudden she didn't want anyone to touch her anymore. She went into a quieter place, and drew on her inner strength. She was clearly in transition. I called the nurse, but she said that she couldn't be in transition yet. Then she wanted to lie down, and she told me that she was pushing. The nurse looked at the strip coming from the monitor, and said that they didn't look like "pushing contractions." The nurse wanted to check her dilation, but my client wasn't even letting the partner or myself touch her at all, even to hold her hand, so having an internal vaginal exam didn't seem like a good idea.

Because of her past, she was very sensitive to people looking at her and touching her "down there." She had asked me to make sure that she was covered, and all day the nurses would pull the blanket off, and I'd put it back over her legs. They'd come in and leave the door open, and I'd go over and quietly shut the door and draw the curtains for her privacy. When the nurse suggested checking her, my client said "no" pretty clearly, but the nurse said the doctor wouldn't come unless they told her how many centimeters dilated the patient was when they called. So, the nurse proceeded to pull off her blanket and reach between her legs, but my client kicked her away, and I replaced the blanket. I was so proud of her for finding her strength and her voice and for sticking up for herself for the first time in her life. I asked her if I could just look without touching, and I saw the baby's hair. I quietly showed the nurse that the baby's head was crowning, and then the nurse finally went to get the doctor.

They said that the doctor was downstairs in a conference, and I asked why she was not running up the stairs. A few more nurses came to move a chair, and bring a bassinet, but nobody was helping my client. When I asked if they could help her, they just kept moving furniture and told her not to push. They said she should just wait for the doctor. She looked up at me and told me mostly with her eyes, but also in words that she needed to push. I told her that this was her birth, and her baby, and that she could push if she wanted to push. I told her that I would not let her baby fall. She had asked me to do perineal support, so I put on gloves and held her tissues as the baby's head came out. I had only been to one vaginal birth before, and it was my own, and so this was the first time that I was really face-to-face with birth. There was a smell that I will never forget (not bad, just different), and it was one of the most challenging moments of my life, but she was so strong and when she looked at me, I just knew what I needed to do. There was no time to procrastinate or to give excuses, I was just there for her, and I held her baby's head in my hands and I made her feel safe enough to push her baby into this world.

As she gave that final push, a pretty distinctive scream came with it, and the midwife in the room next door came in to see if she could help, only to find us with no nurses, and no doctor. I was glad to let her take over, and she suctioned the baby and called the dad to cut the cord. The midwife checked her, but she had no tears to suture. When we reviewed her birth plan, the mom had asked not to hold her baby until she was cleaned up, and so I told the midwife to give the baby to the nurse to get swaddled. But after only a few seconds, the mom wanted to hold her baby, and the delay while they poked and measured seemed too much for her; she wanted her baby so badly. The bond was so strong; it was amazing. She looked so beautiful and so strong in that moment. I took more pictures for her album to save that moment for her forever. Looking at her in that moment, you would not call her a victim. She had her baby in the hospital, but it was just a place. She had worn her own clothes, worked according to her own clock, and pushed out her own baby with no help from a nurse or a doctor.

The next morning, I went to have the pictures printed, and I bought them a pretty album. I am glad to have captured those moments for her to always remember, but I am even happier that I was there with her to help her to find her courage and her voice, and to help ensure that her birth was a source of strength for her as she entered motherhood with this new baby. I was also glad for myself, to learn through my sisterhood with her, that I had my own strength to face my challenges, and that I could use what had happened in my childhood and the intuition that it brought me, to help others.

The Third Trimester

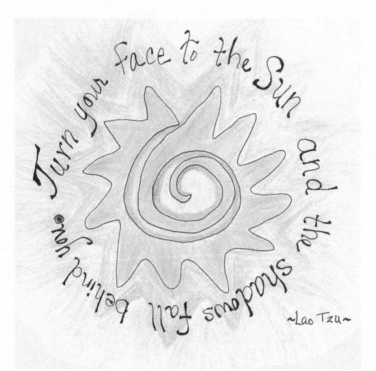

Turn your face to the Sun and the shadows fall behind you.

~Lao Tzu~

Chapter 7: Healing My Wounds, Embracing My Self

I knew that I wanted to have another pregnancy, another birth, and another baby. But I also knew that I wanted to heal my old wounds before I got pregnant again. I spoke to one of the women that had run my doula-training workshop, and she referred me to a family systems therapist. I had never heard of that field, but it turned out to be perfect for me. I had tried traditional "talk therapy" before, but was never happy with it. I'd go in to talk about one problem that was upsetting me, and end up bringing up other memories and then just having even more to be upset about. They would help those hurtful memories to surface, but wouldn't give me the tools to handle the consequences. Like in high school when I was upset because we were reading this horrible story about a girl who is raped and then her baby dies, so I went to the school therapist instead of to English class. Instead of just feeling upset for that girl, he made me remember that I *was* that girl.

He would get me even more upset than going to class, so I just started getting to school late each day instead.

When I went to the therapist who specialized in postpartum depression, she wanted to help me cope with motherhood. The depression doesn't come because motherhood is overwhelming, it occurs postpartum because birth opens up all the parts of yourself that you tried to keep hidden. Labor turns off the logical parts of your brain and makes you *feel* things. Transition brings you to the precipice, and makes you face your true self. Pushing the baby out brings out everything that you had tucked away in those lower chakras. And then those postpartum hormones leave you in a haze, energetically connected to everything in the world, but unable to feel like you have any power to change the world. I told the therapist that I didn't like myself, and I wanted to know if I was supposed to change myself into someone that I could like, or learn to like myself as I was. She told me to take time to meditate, but didn't give me the tools to actually take that step.

I did a lot of preparation before I went to this new family systems therapist. I really wanted to figure out what my questions were, in a way that I could clearly explain them. I needed to be able to articulate the painful memories and then learn to release the power of these wounds to control my life. So, when I started working with her she really helped me to find solutions. She wouldn't just sit there and nod and take notes, she had actual discussions with me. She helped me to make charts and find patterns. She taught me things that challenged my whole belief system, but they made so much sense once I opened myself up to the new ways of thinking.

For the first time, someone actually told me that all the horrible things that happened were not because there was something wrong with me. It was nothing that I did. It wasn't that I wasn't good enough, or didn't try hard enough. I learned that "Victim Energy" could be passed down in families from generation to generation. I had never heard the particulars of the stories, but had always been aware of some deep-seated resentment. There were wounds that were not healed, and then that energy was passed down to me from other women in my family. This thought was so liberating to me, taking the blame off of my shoulders, but it also recommitted me to the healing process, so that I wouldn't pass down this burden to my daughter. I wanted to raise her with love and self-esteem. I wanted to stop perpetuating these negative patterns, destructive body images and self-defeating language.

This idea that there was this energy that was not mine, but was a burden that I carried, made a lot of sense to me once I let it sink in. I'd always felt that I was really a different person inside than the one the world could see. I had always felt this conflict between my true self and the life that I was leading in this body and how I was treated. I found the answer to my question in that if I could rid myself of this negative victim energy, find my true self and embrace and love her, then I could truly heal.

My therapist had explained how a person with abusive tendencies or a power-seeking person can sense a person who has victim energy as soon as they enter the room. When you are with these people you can actually feel them draining your power to increase their own. She never used the term, but afterwards I would also hear them referred to as "energy vampires." I had always wondered "why me?" Why had I been victimized? And it wasn't something that just happened once. It happened over and over, by multiple people. This concept helped to explain the pattern to me, but it was really empowering to think of it as something that I could get rid of, and that I could move on without it.

I started to look into even more fields of alternative healing. I took classes on herbs, aromatherapy, and Reiki for starters. I learned that I was already instinctively doing things to try to heal, in the foods I chose to eat, the perfumed shampoo that I used, and the exercises that made me feel good. The classes reminded me of how much I already knew that had been taught to me since childhood by the women in my family. There were so many traditions that I had not realized were so full of ancient wisdom. In the winter, we make chicken soup with herbs that are anti-inflammatory and break up mucous, which helps us to get through cold and flu season. We take a bath with lavender oils and drink chamomile tea when we need to relax. We drink ginger ale when we have a stomach-ache. We kiss a boo-boo to energetically heal our kids and we instinctively lay our hands on the part of our body that is hurting. Coming from a mainstream background, I had heard so many people speak about herbs and aromatherapy like it was some new-age nonsense, so it helped to tune in to the fact that this was not new at all, it was ancient. Now I could really start to use these tools more purposefully. Without the social stigma clouding my thinking, I really started to pay attention and I started to trust my instincts.

Learning to connect to that ancient wisdom also helped me to start to connect to my body. Focusing on your nutrition and paying attention to how different foods affect you can be a great entry point to learn to tune in to what your body is telling you. Over time I was able to tap in to the wisdom of my pain and other physical symptoms. Dr. Northrup says that the part of the body that is hurting is just trying to teach us something, and we shouldn't try to cure it or to numb it, we need to heal it by listening to it and learning from it. She also says that to heal lower chakra woundings, they need to be witnessed. And I had so many different physical symptoms in my lower chakras! By consciously validating the existence of the wounds, it releases us from their power to control us. I started by journaling, and then, for the first time in my life, I said aloud that I was a victim of sexual abuse.

In her chapter on "Reclaiming the Erotic", Dr. Northrup explains that there is a "sacred spot" deep inside the vagina that stores memories of pain about sexuality, so both arousal and birth can in fact release these memories. (5) This chapter asserts that sexuality is a normal function of life, not just for reproduction, and not just for giving men pleasure so that they'll stick around and help raise the kids. Just as I had before my honeymoon, I worked really hard to visualize sex as something loving and pleasurable. I wanted to view my erotic self as something normal and natural and be able to fight off all my cultural and family belief systems that had taught me to look at it as something dirty and evil.

My husband was more than willing to work with me on trying to grow in this area. He had already spent

8 years of marriage showing me that he would not hurt me and that I could trust him. But sometimes, when it wasn't exactly right and was causing me discomfort, I would just retreat to some other corner of my mind and wait for it to be over instead of speaking up about it. I worked on communicating my feelings and my needs, and tried not to be embarrassed or ashamed about admitting out loud that I had sexual needs and desires. Instead of sex being "okay" or "not too bad," we worked together to make it "great" for both of us.

I must have accessed that "sacred spot" and released some of those personal hurts that I'd kept hidden. I started having increased pelvic pain and ridiculous menstrual cycles. I was "regular," but I would bleed for about 20 out of the 28 days. I even developed sensitivity to the plastics and chemicals in the sanitary pads because I never got much of a break from wearing them. I had all the symptoms of a fibroid and I was scared to get pregnant, but the abdominal ultrasound was completely clear. After a visit to my hometown in which I reconnected with some of those "friends" from my childhood, I had another "episode" of severe and widespread pain. I quit dairy on the midwife's suggestion. I practiced yoga. I wrote and I prayed.

In hindsight, I am thankful that my cycles got so dramatic, because journaling ended up being quite insightful. In *Women's Bodies, Women's Wisdom* I had read about how important all the phases of the menstrual cycle are for your creativity and your intuition. (5) It begins with an inspiration phase with creativity peaking at ovulation, then you enter a reflective time and while you are bleeding you really should rest and tune in to the meaning of things in your life. When I was on the pill for 10 years to regulate my cycles, I also had turned off my intuitive dreams and my creative peaks. When we reframe our cycles as a curse or a disease, we rob ourselves of what really gives women our power. We *do* think differently than men, but it is not a disease; we just live in a society that has schedules and routines that are made to fit in with the ways that men operate. Women can actually be much more productive if they let themselves honor their cycles.

When I started keeping a journal again to mark the phases of my cycles, I also wrote down some of the things that my family was doing, how we were feeling and acting on different days. My daughter was quite challenging at times, and when she was a toddler I had spoken to a pediatrician at a workshop who explained that young girls also cycle, long before they ovulate and begin menstruating. As I charted, I learned to appreciate her cycles. I started to note that when the moon is full, she is caring and affectionate and creative. When it is the dark of the moon though, just let her be. We used to fight and butt heads over little things, but now I just tell her to honor her needs for alone time and I wait for the phase to pass. I am glad that we are practicing this long before the roller coaster of her teenage years begins. We have learned to just blame it on the moon, and then let it go.

And it is not only women who cycle. Men do too. They are a lot more even-keeled and have less dramatic peaks and valleys of emotion than women, but they are not as tough and unemotional as our culture wants them to be. When I reviewed my journal after the first 6 months or so, I noted that my husband was always flattering and expressive in his love at the same time each month. So, if I want him to tell me that I'm beautiful and that he loves me, I just need to wait until it is that phase of his cycle. And then when he hits his busy creative phase he will run around and clean the garage and fix things. That is the time to add something to his list, there is no point in nagging him about it on the wrong week. And then, in his reflective time, he sits down and writes music and plays his guitar for me.

Now, I just need to figure out how to synch our schedules a little better so that when I want to sit and contemplate, he will sit and play me music, instead of running around fixing things. But it is not surprising to me now that when I am putting out creative, positive energy into the world, it is then that he finds that he needs to express how beautiful I am. I am so glad that I had this revelation about my own cycles, and his, because I feel that this level of understanding is what will help us to move through all the stages of parenting and marriage without killing each other.

Parenting in general is not an easy job. It is the hardest job that you will ever do, and there is no time off. Even if I find a substitute to keep my kids safe while I get something else done, I am still a mother. Even if we get out for a rare evening together, we just talk about the kids and how we are going to raise them in this world. We had been labeled so many things by so many people over the years, and in general they were things that we found important, like natural parenting, attachment parenting, breastfeeding, baby-wearing etc. but at the end of the day, we were just trying our best to handle each phase that was thrown at us. Unlike the marketing would have you believe, there is no product that you can buy that will make you the perfect parent. We needed to navigate this world together, with communication and compromise, and at the end of the day know that we had done our best with what we had. And when one phase after another was demanding and exhausting and we felt like the world was against us, it helped to know that we loved each other, and that we were on the same team.

During this time, I also completely changed career paths and started my own business. The hardest part of the adjustment was that my parents wouldn't even talk to me about my new business. They put me down for choosing a career that didn't require all of my degrees and came without a salary. Even writing was something that I was passionate about for years, but my science career was something that I'd been raised to do. My parents had always pushed me towards science. I was good in every subject in school and loved to sing and write poetry. I had always wanted to dance and sing, but had never had lessons. But science was always treated as the noblest career. It was always something I enjoyed and I was good at it, but probably what I liked most was that my parents would always listen to me when I talked to them about my labs. They would always help me with science projects, but it wasn't a priority to come to my concerts.

I have always wanted to help people, wanted to save the world. In school you learn about all these heroes of science. My role models in the family were scientists. My favorite cousin was a biologist. My mother had wanted to be a doctor, but was pushed into lab science instead and then left science to raise us. I went to graduate school and finally had the opportunity to work in the lab of my dreams. But then as I completed my internships, I was exposed to how science works in the real world. It is all based on funding. You cannot just study something because finding the answer would help people to be healthier. Lots of time and money are spent on proving or documenting or quantifying what we already know. There are a few basic things that we need to be healthy, but if there is no money in it, no way to market it, then it gets suppressed. If we were all healthy, how would they be able to sell us pharmaceuticals or do exploratory surgeries? The companies with the money control the research, and the outcomes of the research, to protect their own profits.

I was already starting to become disillusioned, and then I became a mother. I learned that in medical school the doctors did not even have to take one class on nutrition and exercise. Some obstetricians have never seen a natural birth, not even one. They learn medications, and they learn surgical techniques. Why would a woman want to eat right and exercise and be healthy enough to push out her own baby practically for free, when she could pay thousands of dollars for pharmaceuticals and major surgery? Why breastfeed your baby for free and promote their health for their entire lifetime when you can just buy formula and antibiotics, and support the medical field with another lifetime subscription to their services? And don't worry, the government is spending your tax dollars researching diabetes and asthma and obesity, so why promote breastfeeding, which would reduce the incidence of all three?

And breastfeeding is not only important for the baby's health and nutrition; there are numerous benefits for the mother as well. The popular ones are always weight loss and reduction in cancer risk. What about the benefits of stress relief and reduction in depression? What about helping the mother heal from the birth both physically and emotionally? In *Eat, Pray, Love: One Woman's Search for Everything Across Italy, India and Indonesia*, Elizabeth Gilbert explains that yoga poses were originally used so that you wouldn't get stiff from sitting too long in meditation (9). There is even a kind of meditation in which you make it your practice to sit still and not let yourself move, no matter how uncomfortable you get. That reminds me of sitting down to nurse, and you don't dare move and wake the baby that is finally quiet for a moment. How wonderful to be stuck there and have a moment to reflect on the beautiful face of your baby and be thankful for all that you have. I made a "nursing nest" where I would have a few books, the phone, the remote control, a journal and a pen, and snacks and water. That way I was all set and I could nap or get something done, all without losing out on that time that breastfeeding was allowing me to cuddle with my babies, and make that time a priority in my life.

So after reflecting on all the changes in my life and finding the courage to move in a new direction, I applied my educational experience to my work as a birth doula. I helped one family at a time find their way through the medical system. I helped mothers do what they needed to do in order to have safe and empowering births. The goal was not just for them to be grateful for their healthy baby, but to journey into motherhood with their heads held high. Helping those mothers to find their courage and to go to the edge for themselves and their babies helped me to discover my own strength and my own power.

And much as I value this birth work and know that it is necessary, it is hard to be in a field that does not get enough respect in this country. I would work with a woman for weeks or months in preparation, then stay with her for the entire labor. Then, the doctor would come in for the final stages (if at all), and collect a huge fee and all the respect. It is frustrating to live in a society that only values power and money. I had tried to work within the public health system to help families make healthy choices. I had tried to work as a volunteer offering my time and experience to other mothers. I enjoyed my work as a doula, but it is really hard to be on call for births when you have children of your own to care for day and night. I wanted to be able to make my own appointments so that I could put the needs of my family first. And at the end of the day, I needed to do something to generate income without compromising my integrity and my values.

I started my own business, which is much more challenging than any job I have ever done. When you work for yourself, there is no one telling you when or how you need to work. I needed to face rejection and keep going. I needed to keep believing in myself. I needed to believe that I deserved good things. I needed to look my fear in the eye and then follow my dream. My sister encouraged me to go for it and look into what it would take to complete the process. I like to work with families; educating them and helping them work through their own processes to get to their goal. I needed to make that my career and not just my hobby.

It took some time to adjust to my new role. If someone asked what I did, I would say that I was just doing this so that I could make my own hours while the kids are small. Not to say that that wasn't a huge part of taking this chance, but I think in some ways this fits better with who I really am. I like being accountable for my own work. I like doing whatever needs to be done, instead of watching the clock and filling in time with meaningless tasks. At least being my own boss meant being able to bring my kids to my office or work from home with my kids. But trying to concentrate while your kids are demanding your attention is not exactly easy. I know that in facing all of these challenges I am growing much more as a person than if I had retreated back to my old career.

This whole process of transformation would not have been possible without the support of my husband. When I was in high school, my boyfriend worshipped me. It was wonderful at first, but then became smothering. My husband loves me in a much more enduring way. He sees my true self even better than I ever could, and he constantly pushes me to be better and to be happier. He reminds me to focus on him and on others who love me, and try to forget those who are being hurtful, intentionally or not. It is a lesson I would need to keep learning over and over, each time that I found myself working with a difficult client that tested my belief in myself.

By finally saying out loud that I was a victim, I could release the power that it held over me. I could finally believe what my husband had been saying all along. I was worthy of love. I could move forward and take the next step on my journey. I was finally able to look at each challenge as an adventure and a learning experience. Like Gandhi said, I could be the change that I wanted to see in the world.

Chapter 8: Using my Knowledge, Choosing Health

At a BOLD (Birth on Labor Day) grassroots advocacy event in my community, we watched *Birth, A Play* by Karen Brody (10) and then gathered in a festive red tent and created birth art as a form of therapy. I used the pastels and started to draw some circles. I drew a flower with three big petals in the center, one for each of my children. Then I drew circles all around, thinking of all my remaining eggs that could become future children. I shaded in the page with a nice womb-red. I hung the poster on a door where I walked by it every day for the next few months. Even on a hectic, mundane day I could reflect on the feelings that I had had in that sacred space, gathering together with other mothers who understood how I felt about this phase of my life.

One day I left the kids and their noise downstairs with my husband and I went alone to my room to do some yoga. I needed to spend some time in meditation and prayer. A tear slid down my cheek as I put out a call to the universe. I had read a beautiful children's book from the library called *The Mountains of Tibet* in which, at the end of a lifetime, souls could choose to go to heaven or to have another life (11). They could look down and choose which family to join when they were ready. I called out with my spirit to any babies that may want to join my family, and told them that I was ready to welcome one of them.

I started to have all the symptoms of early pregnancy right away. I felt the baby coming to be with me. I was tired and nauseous and having strange dreams. The home pregnancy test was negative. The midwife's test was negative. The blood test at the lab was negative. I didn't understand how that could be. But then the very next month, I felt myself ovulate and then conceive. One day I was on a panel of mothers at a local school for a discussion with teens about pregnancy and birth, and they asked about how soon you could feel that you were pregnant, and another mother spoke about how she had felt the baby's spirit coming to her even before the conception.

This time I had read *all* the books and had gotten to know the local specialists in all different fields of women's health. I had already started to eat nutrient-rich foods and drink Women's Tea with red raspberry leaf to tone my uterus and food herbs to nourish the baby. I went to the chiropractor who used the Webster technique to help align my pelvis and my uterine ligaments to let the baby get into an optimal position. I took the maternal exercise class and learned all the best techniques from the Physical Therapist who specializes in pregnancy and women's health. I breathed deeply and sang to the baby. I told the baby how much it was loved. I made an effort to push the world aside so that I could tune in to my body and this baby and prepare for this birth.

I had hired a midwife as soon as possible because I wanted to have a home birth and there were limited options in my area. I was also due to give birth right at Christmas when all the midwives would want to take time off to be with their families. For the first time in my life, I completely filled out a medical history form. For one thing, my homebirth midwife was the first care provider who had actually asked me about my history. I also knew that it was for her eyes only, and would not be uploaded into some database or kept on file anywhere except in her own office. I also trusted her. I had chosen her because I had heard her telling a birth story in our doula meeting once in which she demonstrated so much love and empathy for the mother, and knew when the mother just needed a little compassion. I knew that she would be the exact presence that I would need during birth and that she would not ask me to do anything that I wasn't comfortable with.

I also asked a good friend to be my doula. She had attended births with my midwife before, and the two of them worked beautifully together. But more importantly, she had become a kind of mother to me over the past few years. When I was younger, I thought it would be great when I grew up, because then my mother and I could be friends. But that didn't happen because she still needed me and leaned on me, but wouldn't reciprocate. And although I always told her that I understood that she had done the best that she could with what she was given, every time I tried to talk to her about how she could offer me support now, she would cry and say that I thought she was a bad mother. So, it was great to have a friend that I could turn to when my own mother couldn't support me in the way that I needed. This friend was one of the only people with whom I never had to pretend. She had a story of her own and had seen it all. I felt that she never judged me and always accepted me as I was.

I also continued to see the midwives at the local birth center so that I could keep a chart there. That way, if I needed to transfer during labor, I could go there instead of having to go to the hospital that doesn't support natural birth at all. During one of my early prenatal appointments I had my children all gathered around me excited to hear the baby, but the midwife couldn't pick up the baby's heartbeat on the Doppler. I tried to act calm while she quickly went down the hall and grabbed the portable ultrasound and then we saw that the baby was fine, but the placenta was low and in front, making it hard to hear the baby. After that I was scared about the placenta growing over my uterine scar. I had just learned a lot about Placenta Accreta because one of my doula clients had that condition and needed to have a surgical birth, so it was on my mind. I was concerned that if the placenta grew into my scar and attached too deeply, I would need to have another surgical birth.

But for the first time, instead of giving in to the worry, I heard the voice of one of the doulas in my head, and I chose to believe in the power of positive thoughts. I sat in a lotus pose and held my hands over my growing uterus. I sent love and energy to my placenta and gently envisioned it moving up and to the back. After doing that for a few weeks, I started to feel movement of the baby down low, where before it had seemed muffled. I was hopeful, but when I went to the 18-week ultrasound I asked about the position of the placenta, and when she said that it was posterior and high, I finally could relax. Some people have told me that the placenta just moves up naturally with the growth of the uterus, but I choose to believe that by having faith and choosing positive thoughts over worry, I helped the change to happen.

I got a copy of *Birthing from Within: An Extra-Ordinary Guide to Childbirth Preparation* by Pam England and Rob Horowitz and I went through some of the reflection exercises with my kids (12). They would draw pictures of what it was like inside the womb. I drew pictures of my three births, the two that I'd experienced and my vision for the coming birth. I had written my stories and I had kept a journal, but having to rely on pictures instead of words opened up some new aspects of the births. When you remember the whole birth, you can tell the story about all the things that happened in chronological time. When I tried to draw the birth, it was all one snapshot of time, but made up of all the images and the range of emotions that I felt. It was the same for the kids who tried to sum up their whole stay in the womb into one feeling.

In the drawing of my first birth I drew a gigantic belly, surrounded by a bunch of faces staring at it. It was from my perspective, looking out over my belly, disconnected from all the different things that were happening while I tried to handle the pain. There were monitors and machines and a surgeon with a scalpel and a menacing stare. The other faces were looking and waiting, but never acting to help me. There was a clock looming, and a big bag of IV solution with Pitocin. Off to the side there was some music and a supportive and loving husband, and a friend, but that gets lost somehow. Possibly the most profound thing that I saw when I reflected on my picture later was that I was not in it.

My second picture shows a bunch of different scenes depicting all the positions that I tried and the parts of the room that we were in at different points in the labor. I have a nice purple, feminine, naked silhouette on the ball, at the ballet bar, dancing with my husband by the window and on all fours in the shower. The pain is there as red streaks coming from my lower back where his head pushed on my spine, but there is pink music everywhere. There is an IV pole there, but it was empty and instead of drugs there is love. And in this picture there is a baby smiling up at me from between my legs, born through a red lotus flower.

My third drawing was my vision for this coming birth. There was a big picture of me taking up almost the whole page. I am wearing a purple sarong and being held by my husband as we danced and he massaged my back and supported my belly with my beautifully hand-woven Guatemalan Rebozo. My mouth is big and red and open, and (because that is how it works) we can assume it is similar down below. There was a rocking chair and a tub and a shower. There were the smiling faces of my children and my sister, and a doula and a midwife (which, with my husband made a circle of seven beautiful souls holding space for the birth). There was a plate of food and drink and fresh flowers. There was a purple belly cast with a spiral spinning into sunshine, and a big pink butterfly to symbolize an empowering transformation.

Around this time I went to a professional conference about cesarean prevention. The speakers were wonderful and there was a great panel discussion. I was sitting at a table with midwives and doctors that I knew, and as the pregnant representative for the table I had to make sure to sit up straight and drink a lot of water and eat a healthy lunch. But despite all of the fascinating epidemiological evidence that was presented about the physical risks and long-term health affects of interfering with birth, I was disappointed to hear dismissive comments from medical professionals who still failed to realize that there are emotional and spiritual aspects of birth. It seemed like some of them do not realize that the woman has an entire life's experience that she brings with her to the birth, and afterwards, the details of that birth will stay with her for the rest of her life. Some of them didn't even seem to realize the *physical* implications of performing major abdominal surgery and that some women have still not completely healed even decades later. The way some of them spoke about surgical birth, you would think that they were talking about a routine trip to the dentist.

The best outcome of the conference was that I met the leader of our local chapter of the International Cesarean Awareness Network (ICAN). She encouraged me to start attending meetings and I am glad that I did. I found other women who (like me) were mourning and healing and trying to understand their births. And many came because they did not want to repeat it the next time. Some were there because they had a friend who had a traumatic birth, and they were looking to do it differently. Each story was different, but the women came together to support each other, to validate each other's feelings, and to help each other to heal. What that means is different to each individual woman. In this group, it is evident that there is not a single, right way to give birth. And we learned that surgical birth can be beautiful and a source of happy memories if it comes from a place of personal power instead of victimization.

During the second trimester, my doula found the book *When Survivors Give Birth: Understanding and Healing the Effects of Early Sexual Abuse on Childbearing Women* by Penny Simkin and Phyllis Klaus at our used bookstore (13). She gave it to me before she even had the chance to read it herself because she sensed that I needed it. The book goes through a series of self-help methods that start with exploring your symptoms to discover what they can tell you about your needs and how to meet them. There were exercises to help you feel emotionally safe, and stress management strategies to ease tension in the body and relax the mind. They gave me self-nurturing activities and grounding techniques to stay fully present and avoid going back and reliving painful memories. And finally, there were ways to break out of the old patterns and beliefs and develop new strategies that didn't include self-damaging behaviors.

Simkin and Klaus use the term "triggers" to refer to something that happens in the present that causes you to react with your negative self-defeating beliefs. After I read this book I rephrased my birth plan to say that I wanted to "avoid the triggers that make me shut down so that I will feel safe and be able to let go, surrounded by positive energy so that I can trust my body." I reflected on my first two births as I'd drawn them and could finally express clearly what my triggers were so that I could avoid them this time. Having been with other women at their births and helping those mothers to identify what it is that they needed helped me to articulate what my needs were.

When I told my VBAC story, even to myself, I would tell about how as the baby came down I let him do it on his own and I didn't want to force it. I was letting the river flow. But when I was finally honest with myself, I could remember how I was ready to push. I was in transition and I was scared, but I knew I was almost there. They thought the water would feel good, so they took my clothes and helped me to the shower. As I sat on the toilet I wondered where my midwife had gone and who this stranger between my legs was. I leaned across the back of the bed and tried to let the baby come down, but the stranger put her hands up in my private area and I couldn't handle that, so I shut down and mentally went someplace else for what ended up being about two hours. Finally, that "ring of fire" brought me back to awareness and she told me that I would have to push him out.

I wrote a list of my triggers and how I could avoid them this time. Because of my childhood, I hate being naked and having people stare at me and make comments. I didn't want to feel watched. I didn't need an audience. That wouldn't be a problem at home anyway, there wouldn't be any strangers randomly opening doors. I don't like to let myself show pain or make noises. I hate the smell of my body. I really wanted to be left alone and preferably under water. I wanted to be able to embrace the sensual nature of birth, but knew that I could never do that with an audience. I wanted caring, loving touch, not invasive touch. I wanted to do my own perineal support and catch my own baby or let my husband help. I knew that when the feelings in my vagina got intense that I would want to retreat. I needed people who understood this and who could help me to stay present. I hate when I feel like I am not being heard. I want the midwife to help *me*, not just my cervix. I wrote it down even though I was confident that this time I had the right midwife and she would take care of me. The midwife who had caught my son is a great person and I really like her now that we've gotten to know each other, but it's too bad we never got to meet before the birth.

I had this perfect vision of how I could have the exact birth that I needed, with loving support in an emotionally safe place. I was so excited to share all this growth from the reflective work that I'd been doing at our next prenatal visit. But as soon as my midwife came in and sat down I knew that something was wrong. She said we had to talk. (We all know what that means.) Because of the political issues in my state, she needed to close her practice and she could no longer attend births. Even worse, she had already called around hoping to find a replacement, but there were no other midwives available on my due date.

My husband looked at me and said that apparently we were going to have to go it alone this time. This was supposed to be our last birth. We'd talked about homebirth throughout the other pregnancies, but being twins and then a VBAC we were nervous. Now we were confident that it was possible for me to push out my own baby. We were just going to have to find our courage.

Part of me liked the idea of just being left alone and catching my own baby. But there was also a bit of fear from all that reading that I had done. I knew that things could go wrong. I also knew that if I was going to be working hard to let myself go into my body and relax and let myself open, I couldn't also stay in my head and coordinate everything. I didn't want to be doing assessments and using science. But I needed to know that everything was under control. I knew that I would reach a point where I'd want someone to tell me everything was fine, and I needed it to be someone else's job to tell me if it was time to go to the birth center. And if I just needed a little help, I didn't want an ambulance to be called and have a bunch of strangers run through the door invading my space and scaring my children.

The worst part was that without the midwife, my doula couldn't come and labor with me. She had decades of experience with birth, and I was sure that she could handle it alone, and that she would be all that I would need, but I legally needed a midwife to be there. I didn't want to pressure her into compromising her credentials by working outside of her scope of practice. I called all around, even to neighboring states, but there was no one available. I asked midwives to come out of retirement. I promised to stay pregnant for an additional month. But there was no one who could come. We hired someone to come and train us in how to use the Doppler and how to assess labor and we bought a birth tub. And I worked on finding my courage.

We researched and planned and got everything in place logistically so that I could feel mentally prepared. We designated a closet for the birth supplies. There were tarps to cover the carpet and towels and yoga mats to put around the tub so that we wouldn't slip and fall. We located the support beam under the floor and moved the furniture so that we could put the tub in the middle of the room. We didn't want to end up with the tub falling through the floor to the basement. My husband was in charge of water hoses and faucet adaptors. We had one hose to fill the tub with clean water, and another to empty the used water out through the window to the lawn. I put a mattress cover under the sheets on my bed just in case, and I bought a set of dark purple sheets. I made a preparation of Comfrey (like a strong tea), and soaked some cloth pantiliners in it and froze them individually on cookie sheets before storing them in freezer bags. Those would feel great on my perineum and help with healing after the birth. We had a whole box of newborn supplies including the hats that the kids had knit on their circular hand looms, and we filled the freezer with casseroles. Having all those things ready helped me to worry a little less and to again turn my focus inward.

I knew that I would have to be strong and healthy and I worked hard to make the birth as easy as possible. I ate healthy food, and drank plenty of water and pregnancy tea. Susun S. Weed says in her book *Wise Woman Herbal for the Childbearing Year* that red raspberry leaf and the nutritional herbs in pregnancy tea can make the birth easier and faster, so I made a quart every morning and drank it throughout the day (14). I saw the chiropractor and went for physical therapy. I wanted to make sure the baby would get into a position that would cause the least amount of complications. I was referred to the website for "Spinning Babies" and I read everything that they had to offer about optimal fetal positioning (15). And then I called a doula friend who does energy work to come and do a healing session with me.

My husband was a great help and took the children out for the evening. We opened the session with a ceremony and then I lay on her massage table in my living room while she worked with my energy. I was amazed that I could feel when it was flowing and when it needed work. I could feel the warmth, even when she didn't physically touch me. But the most profound part was afterwards when I asked her if she could describe to me what she had done.

She said that there was a "sludginess" in my energy. There was energy that was not my own, but that I was carrying. There was a blockage and no energy was going to my sacrum, which was causing my back pain. She restored my energy flow and removed that negative energy that I had been carrying for so long. It felt wonderful to confirm what I had learned at the family systems therapist, and then to do something about it and work towards true healing.

I was already so amazed that she could "read" so much about me from my energy, so I asked her if she could communicate with the baby. I had been so focused on what *I* needed for this birth and for my own healing process. I wanted to know if there was anything that the baby needed from me. The first thing the baby communicated was "to come out, of course." Which I thought sounded just sarcastic enough to fit in well with my family. But the baby also asked for peacefulness, and that sounded good to me.

Then my friend told me that the baby didn't want me to be afraid. I should relax, this was not a new relationship, and that we had known each other before. With tears in my eyes I told her about how strange that was, because just that day I had been thinking about my first baby, the one who didn't come because the time wasn't right. I had called out to all the babies to say that we had room in our hearts for one more. But this wasn't just *another* baby, this was *my* baby who had been waiting for me to be ready, to be healed. And now we could finally be together and have this closure, and this last baby was also my first baby. This time my baby would be born and I would hold them in my arms at last. That hole in my heart was now filled. So, I finally had found what I was searching for, and I knew for sure that we'd do this birth together and that whatever happened, it would be a perfect birth.

My body, My baby, My birth.

-Mb

Chapter 9: Birthing by Myself, but Not Alone

As the last months of my pregnancy approached, my sister worked hard to make sure that I got the Blessing Way that I'd wanted. We got some books out of the library for ideas, and read about different kinds of gatherings on the internet. Neither one of us had ever been to a Blessing Way, but they seemed like such a great idea. Baby Showers are meant to supply you with all the stuff you'll need for the baby, but I already had two or more of everything. I did want to get together with my friends and honor the pregnancy, and bless my belly and my baby. I wanted to really start to let go, and to get ready for the birth. It was a little strange because some of my friends were not aware that I was planning a home birth, and none except my doula was aware that I was planning to birth on my own. At the end of the day though, a Blessing Way is just a nice way to mark the occasion, and everyone loves a celebration.

I didn't ask my mother to come, because she had

been so depressed lately and I didn't want to be drained by that negative energy at that important time. I wanted the day to be focused on me and on the baby, but it broke my heart that I couldn't share this with her. Every time I tried to talk to her about my first birth, she would just get angry and put all the blame on the midwife. But we had both known that the medical system was broken and I had brought her there to take care of me and to protect me. She had let me down, and while I understood and I forgave her, the hurt was still there. My therapist had finally helped me to realize that my mother has never protected me; she has never known how. I had thought that her experience with birth and breastfeeding would come in helpful. I would always call her when I was worried about something, and she would give me the technical information, but that was all she had to give. Because of her past and her own issues, she cannot give me the nurturing that I need. I sometimes feel like she cannot see who I really am, and can't hear me when I cry for help. So for this birth, I realized that I couldn't rely on her. I was afraid that she would let me down again and I knew that it would break my heart so I tried to just create distance to protect myself from that hurt. But the distance hurt, too. We later told her that the Blessing Way was a last minute thing, but I think she knew that there was more to it than that.

We did plan the gathering for when my sister-in-law and my brother were in town, and it turned out to be a great idea. My sister-in-law was great and really helped my sister with the planning and the final preparations. I had always ended up doing a lot of the preparation for my own bridal and baby showers. When I got married, my sister was a young teenager, and so I ended up doing most of the planning. I hosted my baby shower in my house and needed to do a lot of the work to get ready. So, this time it was a real treat to let them care for me and handle all the details after I gave them my input on what aspects were most important to me. It was that letting go that was exactly what I needed.

In the invitation, they had asked the women to bring an inspirational poem or saying, and a bead that held some meaning. They were asked to bring small gifts that would be a treat for me in the last weeks of pregnancy, like chocolates or bubble bath. We found silver beads that said "Believe" and that became our theme. We made friendship bracelets out of embroidery floss (and attached the bead) for the women to wear as a reminder to think of me until I gave birth, and then they could cut them off. I felt that if I knew all these women believed that I could do it, and were supporting me and praying for me and sending me positive energy, then I could also "believe" in myself.

The morning of the Blessing Way my sister drew some birth art (that I would later use for this book) and then had me sit and color in the pictures while they cleaned my house and prepared all the food. My sister-in-law made a beautiful cake with a gloriously pregnant purple woman on it. It even had edible silver beads! Then they prepared a bubble bath for me and sent me off to relax while they got everything ready. I got dressed and came down the stairs to find candlelight and fresh flowers and my birth art decorations hanging from colorful ribbons. The room was so pretty; I ended up keeping it that way for months. My husband had taken the boys out to a friend's house and my daughter was invited to stay with us women. I am really glad that she chose to be a part of my special day, and I am glad to have given her a positive image of sisterhood.

After my friends arrived and we visited for a while, we sat in a circle and they shared the meaning of the beads that they had each brought, and they shared their poem or saying. It was so beautiful it made me teary-eyed. They sat me in the rocker and my doula washed my feet and massaged them with oil. Since I was then stuck in the chair, I had to let my friends serve me food and bring me drinks. Then I let them see my belly, with all its stretch marks and scars from where it had torn, and they drew designs on it with henna. It was hard to be so vulnerable, but we had created an atmosphere where I felt safe and loved.

We listened to "Returning" by Jennifer Berezan (16), which had been introduced to me by my yoga teacher, and it was perfect for birth. It is a beautiful chant to the Mother of Us All that was recorded in an ancient underground temple. The songs were stuck in my head, and as I drove in my car or waited for the school bus I would improvise my own verses.

"Returning, Returning, Returning…"

…to a quiet place

…to a warm embrace

…to your lover's arms

…to your body's strength

…to a childlike grace

…to your one true self

…to a peaceful time

That night, we sat in the living room by firelight and candlelight, and my husband played his guitar while everyone worked on artistic projects. My brother helped my sister put my beads on a necklace and I drew a picture of each bead and wrote down who brought it and what it meant. My sister-in-law was making me pages for a scrapbook, and before she left that weekend I had a beautiful keepsake to share (unlike those baby books that I promise I will work on after they all leave for college). I sat in the rocking chair and worked on crocheting the baby blanket. I wanted to keep that feeling with me, and I stayed on that romantic "cloud 9" for the rest of the pregnancy.

Meeting with my doula and going for a pregnancy massage also helped me to stay in my body. I also made a belly cast. I almost passed out from trying to look down while my husband laid the plaster cast strips on my belly, but he threw the window open and let in the cold air just in time. I was no longer sitting up as straight as I had wanted and when I slumped over I squished the plaster, but I did not end up ruining the belly cast entirely. After it dried, it was a great project to keep me busy for the last weeks of the pregnancy. Whenever I didn't know what to do with myself, I would sit and sand the cast, moving my hands in circles over the belly and the breasts, and then put on another layer of drywall plaster and sand it again. When I had it pretty smooth I sealed it and added coats of paint. I painted it purple and put the spiral with the sunshine around it, just like I had been drawing the whole pregnancy as I doodled with the kids and on my birth art for my Blessing Way.

Doing an artistic, physical project kept me in my body, but as I manually worked on creating my belly cast I could also mentally prepare for the upcoming birth. I focused on my birth vision and I recited my mantras and I sang songs that helped me to surrender and to let go. I needed to let go of my expectations, my worry, and all of that guilt and shame that had been weighing me down for far too long.

I asked my doula if she thought that I was being naïve to feel so confident that everything was going to be fine…better than fine, it was going to be perfect. But I felt like I really deserved this birth after all that this baby and I had already been through. I was almost 16 the first time I tried with this baby, and after learning and growing for another 16 years, I really believed that this was our time to finally get it right. All those other challenges that I had gone through were not just my stories; they were from the victim energy that I carried for all those women in my family who could not heal their wounds. I had carried it long enough. I would heal for them, and for my children and myself. I would break those chains. This was my time, with this baby, and I deserved good things.

At the end of each day I would fall asleep holding my belly and feeling how it had changed since the day before. Each night I would connect with my baby in my dreams. In each of my pregnancies I had seen the babies in my dreams, and I had always felt confident that I knew them so well before they were born. This time I was having really vivid dreams about a beautiful, bold daughter and I pictured her so clearly and I had dreams about her becoming a visionary and a leader. I had never found out the sex of my babies before the birth, but I had been right about each of them so far so I should be confident in believing my dreams, but somehow I kept thinking something didn't make sense. I kept second-guessing myself and I even considered having an ultrasound, but I wanted to stay in tune to my intuitions instead of relying on technology to get to know the baby. Whatever it was that was bothering me, I knew that I just had to have faith.

We set off on our last family trip before the birth, traveling to Thanksgiving Dinner at the in-laws'. Car trips are perfect for long, philosophical conversations because for those few hours we can't do other projects; we just sit with each other and talk while the children sleep, secure in their car seats. I explained to my husband the energy session that I'd had, and how profound it was. I shared with him my new confidence that everything would be just fine. I figured that this baby had already been through enough to be here with us, and this time it was meant to be perfect. We had found our courage to birth by ourselves if need be, but I still didn't want to be alone. I wanted nurturing. I wanted my doula, and I wanted my midwife to look at me with love and care in her eyes, and I wanted to share the moment with women that I knew truly understood the meaning of it all.

My midwife had gone out of town for a few weeks and I hoped that she'd had the time that she needed to process what I knew must be a very difficult situation for her. I had called her right before our trip and I asked her to think about coming to my house on the day of my birth, just to be there. I told her that she could just happen to stop by as a friend, and maybe hang out in the other room and work on her knitting or something. I knew that just having her energy and her presence in my house would be enough. And if anything did happen, she would be there to tell me what I needed to do. She didn't say anything, but I asked her to think about it and we'd talk the following week.

One other not so small detail that I'd been trying to avoid worrying about, and that I didn't happen to mention to my midwife, was that the baby had turned to the breech presentation. I had felt the baby turn earlier in the week, and when I palpated my belly I knew the baby's bottom should not flex like a neck, but I kept denying it. I'd gone for a prenatal appointment at the birth center right before the trip, and the nurse-midwife there said "are you sure the baby is head down?" In saying that she confirmed what I had known but hadn't acknowledged. So, when we got to my in-laws' house I went upstairs and laid upside down with my butt up on a pile of pillows in a breech-tilt and I cried. All night long I pushed on the baby and encouraged it to flip over. In the morning I called my doula and I cried. She said that babies turn to the breech position when something is unsettling. She also said that I needed to stop pushing on the baby since I was starting to have contractions and the last thing I wanted was to have the baby too early at a hospital away from home. What I really needed was to finally sort out my birth plan.

The next morning as the children played with toys and put together puzzles on the floor, my husband started to pluck the strings of his guitar. It was the most beautiful tune I had ever heard, and totally different from how he usually strums the guitar. The song was slow and meditative and he scribbled some lyrics in his notebook and then began to sing. I sat there and cried when I heard the lyrics that were the exact expressions of my heart, that I had never been able to put into words so well. That song was the perfect birth plan and it told me that despite everything else he may say or do, my husband understood completely on a deeper level, and we were in this together.

The funny part was thinking about how all this

must have looked to the rest of the family. They had no idea that we were planning a homebirth, never mind that I was in the last month of the pregnancy with no guaranteed care providers. But they didn't even know that the birth was so close, since I wouldn't tell any of them a due date. I told them the baby would come when it was ready, most likely in the winter, probably in the new year. They didn't understand. They kept asking me why the doctors couldn't figure out an actual due date. That made it even funnier, because I hadn't seen a single doctor the whole pregnancy. The midwives had given me a due date though, and I just wasn't sharing, since my family had lost the privilege of having that information after making me crazy during the final weeks of my other pregnancies, which went longer than they expected. I was joking about it to my husband at one point, and then he mentioned that I hadn't even told him the actual due date!

So there we were, doing breech tilts and singing songs about unassisted homebirth, all in the middle of this group of people that we were related to, but who didn't seem to understand us at all. To them, there was nothing to plan for. When you feel something, you go to the hospital, they turn off the feelings, and then the doctor delivers the baby. No preparation needed. Even our friends who supported homebirth did not support free-birthing, so we were starting to really feel like we were going it alone.

When we went home I called my doula to check in and tell her that everything was fine. The baby had turned, no doubt because of the power of that amazing song. I went to the chiropractor and had my pelvis aligned, and the baby dropped a few inches, deep into my pelvis, head down, to turn no more. My doula called a few days later and said that she had seen my midwife at a party. They got to talking and she had said, "You know, I might have a knitting project to do after all." So everything was finally starting to come together at almost 38 weeks. I had found the courage to do this myself, but I would not have to do it alone.

Every evening after that, I would sit in my rocking chair after I put the kids to bed, and I would stroke my belly while the contractions came every few minutes. My doula called it the "installment plan." I would labor a little each night, softening, ripening, and getting ready. In the quiet house after my husband and my sister went to sleep, the contractions would get going pretty strong. I'd stand naked in front of the bathroom mirror in the moonlight and rub my belly and tell the baby that I was ready if this was the time, but not to hurry for me. I practiced letting go. I let myself feel everything, and not try to avoid or stop the process. Usually I just use the mirror to look for any imperfections that need correction, but I do not see my whole self. I had always hated mirrors (and pictures of myself). So I practiced seeing myself. I practiced loving myself. Then when I got too tired, I'd lay down to rest and then the next thing I knew I'd wake up in the morning, still pregnant.

One night two weeks later, I stayed up late taking pictures of my naked belly and breasts, somehow knowing that this was my last chance. That night I had a dream that my water released. I'd always wanted it to happen on its own and not with an amni-hook, so I was surprised to find that when I got up my pajamas were actually wet and it wasn't just a dream. I got up and changed my clothes and put on a pad and put a towel on the bed. It was 2:30 in the morning. I woke up my husband to tell him. I was so excited. I was crying and kissing him. I was so relieved that I had actually been able to release and "let it go." I asked my husband if he was ready to have another baby. He said that he had to go to work in the morning, and then he went back to sleep. I got up. I was too excited to sleep. I made jars of tea, bottles with water and lemon juice and energy drinks. I ate yogurt and listened to the baby's heartbeats with my fetoscope. I started cleaning and made a pot of soup. I gradually started to turn the heat up in the house.

Then I lay back down to rest, and when I woke up,

my husband was gone. I could not believe that he had actually gone to work. I called my doula and she was at another birth. The kids were home from preschool and Kindergarten for the week and were fighting over every little thing as usual. So my sister and I made cookies and did craft projects with the kids and then bundled them up and sent them outside to play in the snow. They made me a snow-woman with a big spiral belly. The contractions spaced out a little while we were busy, but they never stopped. After lunch I had three really strong contractions right on top of each other, so I filled the birth tub halfway just in case.

My husband finally came home after taking his time and stopping to finish his Christmas shopping. I thought we could finally focus on the labor but he was actually trying to get me to talk about paying the bills and sorting the paperwork. We have a picture of him in his suit and tie next to me in my tie-dye nightshirt breathing through a contraction while sitting on the birth ball. Then we were into the dinner and bedtime routine. After the kids were in bed we finished filling the pool, and my doula came over. My husband played his guitar and we had a nice social visit. We played with some litmus paper to confirm that I was leaking amniotic fluid and we listened to the baby. But it felt like everyone was waiting for me to perform. So I sent my doula home to see her family since she'd been gone at a birth all day and her son was just coming home from college. I thought we'd send my sister to bed so that we could have some alone time, but my husband had rented a movie, so he put that on, and then he fell asleep while I tried to relax. When I laid down on the couch, the baby got jumpy, so I had my husband get the Doppler and count the heartbeats. The number was low, 114 beats per minute instead of in the 130s where it had been all day, and I was worried. My husband methodically wrote it in the notebook and then casually went to bed and left me alone freaking out about what to do. Finally, after changing positions a few times, the baby seemed happier and I listened again, and it was back in the normal range.

I tried to sleep but I was too angry. Then when I was almost relaxed, I heard a hissing sound and I jumped up to find the cat on the edge of the inflatable pool where he had punctured it with his claw. I was so mad, I ran to get the vinyl repair kit and I fixed the leak and sent the cat outside in the snow. After that, I was determined to use that pool, and I was not at all sleepy. So I set to work boiling pots of water to add to the water in the pool and I eventually got the water up to temperature. I had built a tent around the pool out of the kids' fort building kit and my purple tapestries from college so that I could lay in there naked and if someone walked into the room I'd still have my privacy. I put on my "Returning" CD and got in the pool and the water felt so nice and it started to ease some of my frustration. I rubbed my belly in big circles and I talked to the baby and then the contractions started coming really strong.

I tried to relax and just let the baby come. I kind of thought that it would be great to just have the baby born there quietly, and then when everyone woke up they'd find the baby was already born. But the labor was strong and I was getting anxious. And then the pool got cold. I couldn't be in the kitchen heating the water in pots on the stove and float in the water and relax at the same time. I should've bought the submersible heater, but it was too late for "should've." I woke up my husband to put him on water duty. He doesn't do too well when awoken from a deep sleep, so we had a quick fight, but then he listened to the baby and wrote the heart rate in the notebook.

At this point, I knew that it was almost time for the children to wake up and come looking for their breakfast. I had finally gotten into a groove and labor was coming fast now. I was breathing hard and swearing at my husband, and I didn't want to lose momentum when the kids came downstairs. I asked him to call my doula so that she could stay with me while he tended to their needs. He didn't want to wake her, but I knew that once she saw that the sun was already out she'd wonder what was going on since she had planned to come back in the middle of the night. After I asked about half a dozen times (starting off sweetly and politely, of course, but with my voice gradually increasing in volume and pitch), he finally called my doula and said that "nothing was happening," and told her that she could stop by later (if she wanted). When I overheard him say that, I could've killed him. Luckily she knew better and arrived a few minutes later like I knew that she would.

After the long night that I'd spent hauling pots of water and laboring alone, I was exhausted. I slept a little on the couch while my doula rubbed my tired legs with some Arnica lotion. My oldest son brought me a cool cloth and rubbed my back. The kids took turns bringing me a drink. My daughter drew me pictures. I liked that they could come and go as they felt comfortable. I knew that my sister was taking good care of them, and so I was able to focus on the labor.

When the head hit my sacrum I was so glad to have my doula there to provide counter-pressure, and more importantly, emotional support. She had already called my midwife who had said that she'd come right over. After we hung up the phone, I had felt a strange pop. The baby's head had plunged down the last little bit and I was already pushing when the midwife got there. I used a technique we'd practiced in my pregnancy exercise class in which you make an "S" sound while you exhale, which uses more efficient muscles by pulling in your lower belly compared to an "O" sound which pushes out your mid-belly. If you try both, you can feel how the different muscles engage and how you can focus your efforts to help the pushing stage move along more quickly.

At this point we had taken the tapestries down from around the pool so that my doula and midwife could help if I needed anything. I was back in the pool and I was wearing a dark red cotton tank dress, which was comfortable even underwater, and it gave me the confidence and the privacy that I needed, and it matched my toenails! I was also wearing my birth necklace with the beads from my Blessing Way and my "Believe" bracelet.

I just remember looking up and seeing the midwife's smiling face from across the pool, and I knew that I could do it. And she was wearing dark purple. Perfect. She asked how far I had to go, and I said that I didn't know. She told me how to check, and when I put my finger in, the head was two knuckles away...then only one. That was the extent of all my assessments.

When the baby crowned I reached down and provided my own perineal support. I could feel the head coming through while I held my tissue back so it wouldn't tear. I had done this for other women at their births because they had asked me, but it still took courage for me to do this with my own body and with people there watching and taking pictures. But it really helped to feel myself stretching and feel that it was a baby causing the strong feelings. I could feel when I needed to relax and when I needed to push further. I felt like I was tearing at the bottom where I'd healed from the stitching after my last birth, and I didn't have enough hands. I asked my doula to hold it there, and she just gave me a little extra support with a folded washcloth and she kept asking me if what she was doing was okay. My husband was leaning over the side of the pool and holding me in his arms with one hand on my head, and one on the baby's.

I kept telling myself to stay present to the task at hand, and I *let go*. The head pushed out and I could feel an ear. That ear made the fact that this was my baby so real that I became excited instead of getting scared because the burning feeling in my vagina and my vulva was so intense. I pushed past the burning and I pushed the body out and brought the baby to my chest. Everyone from my initial drawing that I had made to represent my birth vision was in the room, and my baby and I were surrounded by love and support. Caroline Myss teaches about the importance of the number seven: the seven stages of healing, the seven chakras, the seven sacraments, and the seven sacred truths (6). Here I was, surrounded by seven powerful, loving and beautiful souls, with all that amazing energy focused on my baby and me for this birth. And the baby had gotten the peaceful birth that had been requested, and most importantly, had *come out*.

We wrapped the baby in warm, purple towels and put purple sheets over the couch. After I stood up and delivered the placenta into a bowl, I put on a dry nightgown and we snuggled on the couch and nursed. And as we lay there, bonding and falling in love, I tried to figure out how it had happened. As soon as the baby was out, I had seen it. Yes, there was definitely a penis. A part of me had known that it would be there, had sensed that this baby was a boy. But I had felt all along that I was supposed to give birth to a girl, that there was a daughter that needed to be born. We had the name chosen that would best represent a daughter who was strong and beautiful unto herself, and loved for who she was inside. No pale, shrinking violet. So, although I had had the perfect birth, and a perfect and beautiful baby, I couldn't help but wonder, "Where is Magdalena?"

I had worked so hard to let go and to let my body give birth, while truly staying present to the process and not hiding from it. But now I had to come to terms with the fact that this phase was over. This was my last pregnancy, my last birth, my last baby. As I fell in love with my son (or more accurately, kept noticing in new ways how much I had loved him all along), I cried about all the cute little dresses as I took them off of their hangers in the closet and gently folded them. My eyes would tear up as I put away each size of baby clothes for the last time, knowing that my daughter would not have a little sister. I grieved over having to close that chapter of my life.

In those wonderful early weeks, snuggled up with my baby that had taken 16 years to hold in my arms, I felt complete and whole at last. I wanted to freeze time and stay in that magical state forever. The rest of the world was going about business as usual, but I was so different. Why couldn't anyone see that? Why couldn't they sense that this is the most important thing in the world? How can everyone worry about money and filing their taxes and meeting arbitrary deadlines when there is something so much more important? What would I do when the postpartum hormones wore off and the real world crept back in; when I was back in the world of ordinary things instead of floating through that world of miracles? I wanted to stay in that moment, in that warm and soft and dimly lit space, with gentle movement and beautiful music and angels in the gently falling snow. I wanted everything to stay all sparkly and colorful. I wanted to hide behind my purple tapestry that protected me from the world of ordinary days, of work and running a household and the demands of everyday things. I just wanted to stay beyond the veil and to feel that a little longer.

And now as I sit here all snuggled up with my baby in my nursing nest, typing one-handed while the baby sleeps on my other arm, and trying to make sense of it all, I realize that this is not the end, but another beginning.

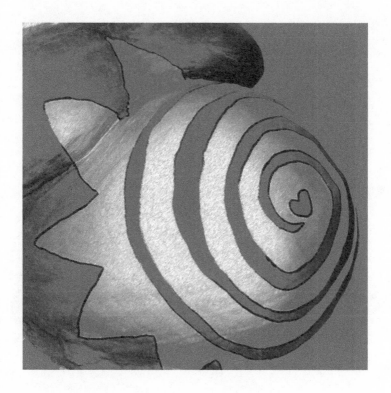

Epilogue: The Birth of Magdalena

In the months following my third and final birth, I planned a special ceremony for my family. We had waited for winter to pass before we could bury the placenta in the yard, and I wanted to plant a special tree after the spring thaw. Each of the children had a tree that we had planted when they were babies, but we had never been able to keep one of the placentas. I couldn't just let this sacred moment pass. My doula and my midwife came over when the baby was six months old and the ground was warm again, and we lit candles and incense. I told the story of my three births and how I was so enriched and fulfilled as the mother to these four amazing children. I said aloud how glad I was to have had these babies, with this man, and how they had all filled the hole that was in my heart.

As I gave each person a spiral charm I explained how I had been drawing spirals inside the shape of a sun when I colored with the kids and how I was drawn to that image long before I understood that it was an ancient symbol with deep meanings in many cultures. I had colored it on the driveway with chalk and sculpted it with play dough. I had made the same design on my belly with henna at my Blessing Way, and I painted it on my belly cast. Then my doula had spiraled the umbilical cord on top of the placenta before we packaged it up to put it in the freezer. From many internet searches, I had come to find that the spiral represents fertility, birth, transformation, growth, the soul and expansion. It also represents an inner journey to the center of one's soul. The spiral is also associated with water and power, which is a great description of my final birth. A clockwise spiral is also used to represent the winter sun that was shining on me that day. I was so glad to welcome him with all my children surrounding me; and with only loving, supportive, beautiful souls in the room. I was so glad to have given birth entirely from my own power, reclaiming my body and my self as my own.

As we buried the placenta I said: "I am burying this placenta as part of my womb where all my babies grew." Then we planted the tree. I had been trying to find the perfect tree and had finally happened upon a Spiral Willow when visiting my extended family. How perfect? I brought a cutting home and had been rooting it in a jar before this planting. At that point in the ceremony, I gave each child a dark, red rose that I had cut from the bushes that grow along the path and said to them: "My belly has expanded and contracted over these past years. I have held all four of you in my belly, and in my arms, and I will always hold you in my heart." They each put a rose around the baby tree and then went to hang their spiral charms from their own trees.

I then walked inside with my midwife and my doula and they laid me on my colorful Mayan Rebozo and performed the Womb-Closing ceremony. With one of them on each side, surrounding me with love and support yet again, they wrapped the shawl tightly around me and held it firmly to the ground. We thanked my womb and blessed it, resealing it as a private, inward space, only for me. I accepted my womb as the source of my creativity and thought of all the good things that I could still create in the world. I reflected on the person that I had become.

Since the birth I had already noticed some changes in myself:

- I felt that I deserved good things.
- I believed that my body was strong and healthy and capable.

- I believed that I was beautiful, and I let people see me.

- I could be hurt or disappointed, but not take it personally and not be thrown into a deep depression.

- I could place blame within others when it was something that was their issue, not mine. It wasn't that I didn't deserve to be loved, or to be heard, or to be seen. If they could not see the true me, it was *not* because I was invisible, it was because they were blind.

- I was a *survivor*, not a victim.

This ceremony helped me to reflect on the whole process of becoming a woman and giving birth. Even though from the start I thought that I believed in the transformative power of birth for women, it took me three tries to really *feel* it. I had believed it to be true when I read about it, but I didn't have true faith in it. I didn't need to understand it with my head; I needed to feel it in my body and in my soul. In our culture, women are taught to fear and deny their own power throughout their life, and then it becomes hard to draw on that power when it is time to give birth. Each time that women start to reclaim birth, the medical system finds more ways to control birth and strip it of its meaning and thus deny us our power even further. I imagine a world where our daughters love themselves and their bodies and where our sons can love strong and powerful women and are in awe of what they can do.

In *Anatomy of the Spirit*, Caroline Myss tells us that "Self Esteem and conscious personal power sometimes develop at a memorable point in life that signifies an initiation into spiritual adulthood" (6). For me, that moment was reached through my three births as a rite of passage. The lessons that birth needed to teach me were complex, and it was a long journey. Dr. Myss teaches about the four stages through which we progress. My first (surgical) birth was the "revolution" that awoke me to the flaws in our society and helped me to realize that I needed to establish my own sense of authority. My second (VBAC) birth helped me towards "involution" in which I needed to explore my interior self and my life's purpose. The self-knowledge was painful and hard to face at times, but in the end was very healing. She calls the third stage "narcissism" in which you redefine yourself to suit your own beliefs, not those of your family or your society. My third birth at home helped me to develop a strong sense of self. Myss says it is okay if the fourth stage becomes a long journey and she calls it "evolution." Going forth from this stage of my life, I would need to maintain my faith and stay true to the self that I had worked so hard to discover and to embrace.

As I lay there wrapped in my Rebozo and let myself be cared for yet again by these beautiful and strong women, I thought of the Gloria Steinem quote in *Revolution from Within (7)*. She said, "I didn't know how to be a daughter and accept help and nurturance, though I wanted them desperately." And then I knew that I could finally let myself be the "*daughter*" that I had always needed to be. In the end, giving birth wasn't just about becoming a mother; it was about letting me be a daughter.

I have come around another turn of the spiral. "When I turn my face to the sun, the darkness falls behind me" (Lao Tzu). I have finally found my true self, the woman within. *I* am the strong, beautiful daughter that I was seeking. *I* am the girl that needed to be born.

I am Magdalena.

References

1. *The American Way of Birth* by Jessica Mitford. Diane Publishing Company (1999) ISBN 0788163450

2. *Thank You, Dr. Lamaze - A Mother's Experiences in Painless Childbirth* by Marjorie Karmel Doubleday (1965) ASIN: B000KNZPMK

3. "Don't Push the River, It Flows by Itself" by Laura Shanley (An Excerpt from her book *Unassisted Homebirth*) Available at URL: http://www.unassistedchildbirth.com/inspired/river.html

4. *Gift From the Sea: 50th Anniversary Edition* by Anne Morrow Lindbergh. Pantheon Books (2005) ISBN 9780679732419

5. *Women's Bodies, Women's Wisdom: Creating Physical and Emotional Health and Healing* by Christiane Northrup, MD Bantam Books (1998) ASIN B000RJ0D1A

6. *Anatomy of the Spirit: The Seven Stages of Power and Healing* by Caroline Myss. Three Rivers Press (1997) ISBN 9780609800140

7.   *Revolution from Within: A Book of Self-Esteem* by Gloria Steinem. Little, Brown and Company (1993) ISBN 9780316812474

8. *Touching, The Human Significance of the Skin* by Ashley Montagu. Harper & Row (1978) ISBN 0060129794

9. *Eat, Pray, Love: One Woman's Search for Everything Across Italy, India and Indonesia* by Elizabeth Gilbert. Penguin (2007) ISBN: 9780143038412

10. *Birth, A Play and BOLD Red Tents by Karen Brody (2011) http://www.birththeplay.org/*

11. *The Mountains of Tibet* by Mordicai Gerstein. Harper Collins (1989) ISBN 0064432114

12. *Birthing from Within: An Extra-Ordinary Guide to Childbirth Preparation* by Pam England and Rob Horowitz. Partera Press (1998). ISBN 0965987302

13. *When Survivors Give Birth: Understanding and Healing the Effects of Early Sexual Abuse on Childbearing Women* by Penny Simkin and Phyllis Klaus. Classic Day Publishing (2004). ISBN 1594040222

14. *Wise Woman Herbal for the Childbearing Year*

by Susun S. Weed. Ash Tree Publishing (1986) ISBN 0096746000

15. *SpinningBabies.com -Easier Childbirth through Fetal Positioning* by Gail Tully. Maternity House Publishing (2008)

16. "Returning" by Jennifer Berezan. Edge of Wonder (2001) ASIN: B00005NC32 Audio CD

One Final Note

And an additional note of recognition to Elizabeth Gilbert and her book *Eat, Pray, Love* for introducing me to the Sanskrit word "antevasin," meaning "one who lives at the border" or someone who is in-between worlds. It describes someone who is in the world, but not of the world; someone who is a spiritual seeker. When I first read the description of this word, I felt like there was finally one word that could explain so much about who I really am.

About the Author

M.B. (Michelle) Antevasin is a mother, a teacher, and a healer and she works at the intersection of science and spirituality to break patterns and promote healing. Michelle has been studying the science of Health and Wellness for over twenty years. She has a Bachelor's degree in Biology and a Masters of Public Health in Epidemiology and is a Certified Science Teacher.

While raising her 4 children she became an accredited La Leche League Leader and a Professionally Trained Birth Doula and recently completed a 3-year Energy Healing training and is a Certified Family Trauma Professional. She currently runs her own health consultation business and is a Professor of Business, Health and Science. She volunteers with Children and Families in her community and she works to end patterns of abuse and trauma by sharing her own healing journey through her writing and she brings to her classes and workshops her experience as a teacher, a mother, a survivor and a healer. Michelle also holds support groups monthly and is available for private healing sessions.